Personalized Therapy for Multiple Myeloma

Saad Z. Usmani • Ajay K. Nooka

Editors

Personalized Therapy for Multiple Myeloma

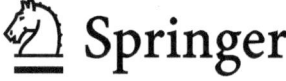 Springer

Editors
Saad Z. Usmani
Department of Hematologic
 Oncology and Blood
Levine Cancer Institute
Charlotte, North Carolina
USA

Ajay K. Nooka
Department of Hematology and Oncology
Winship Cancer Institute
 of Emory University
Atlanta, Georgia
USA

ISBN 978-3-319-61871-5   ISBN 978-3-319-61872-2   (eBook)
https://doi.org/10.1007/978-3-319-61872-2

Library of Congress Control Number: 2017951926

Printed on acid-free paper

This Springer imprint is published by Springer Nature
The registered company is Springer International Publishing AG
The registered company address is: Gewerbestrasse 11, 6330 Cham, Switzerland

This book is dedicated to our patients, their caregivers, and our families.

Preface

The management of multiple myeloma (MM) has evolved tremendously over the last decade, from being an orphan disease with limited treatment options to a disease that can be chronically managed for most patients. The knowledge of the heterogenous disease biology and development of novel drug classes (immunomodulatory drugs, proteasome inhibitors, etc.) that target this disease have resulted in more than doubling the overall survival for MM patients. There is a recognition that MM has several different molecular/clinical phenotypes and that several genomic subclones exist in any given patient—clearly, MM is not a one-pathway disease. Given such variability, a cookie-cutter approach may not be applicable to MM, and many factors influence treatment strategies for a given patient. Several long-standing paradigms are being shifted, and such changes are coming at a rapid pace.

We know that monoclonal gammopathy of undetermined significance (MGUS) gives rise to smoldering and active MM yet had previously been unable to identify the subset that is at the highest risk of progression to active disease. By utilizing clinical variables, flow cytometry, novel imaging techniques, and genomic tools, there are models that can help identify this "high-risk" group. Clinical trials are now evaluating the role of early therapeutic intervention in this group. For newly diagnosed MM, better prognostication models are being developed that include biologic data. Novel agent regimens are starting to look beyond the proteasome inhibitor/immunomodulatory drug induction regimens, incorporating new mechanisms of action and strategies. Autologous stem cell transplants remain an important part of early therapy, but investigations are under way to examine the timing of this modality. Gone are the days when fixed duration (as is the case of solid tumors) was the norm in MM, as maintenance therapy has shown to improve survival outcomes and has become a standard of care. Several three-drug regimens have shown to be more effective than two-drug regimens for both newly diagnosed and relapsed MM patients in large phase III trials, thus laying rest to the debate and confirming what we would have intuitively guessed based on MM biologic heterogeneity. MM is becoming a chronically managed disease where supportive care measures, pain management, and bone health management become an integral part of improving patients' quality of life. Yet, there remain many research questions that remain unanswered, and the task of curing this cancer is not accomplished.

In this book, we have attempted to provide an assimilation of the most current data in advising the clinicians on the practical management of MM patients written by the foremost authorities in the field.

Charlotte, NC   Saad Z. Usmani
Atlanta, GA   Ajay K. Nooka

Contents

Risk Stratification in Newly Diagnosed Smoldering Multiple Myeloma

María-Victoria Mateos and Jesús San-Miguel

1.1 Introduction

Smoldering multiple myeloma (SMM) is an asymptomatic plasma cell disorder defined in 1980 by Kyle and Greipp on the basis of a series of six patients who met the criteria for multiple myeloma (MM) but whose disease did not have an aggressive course [1].

At the end of 2014, the International Myeloma Working Group (IMWG) updated the definition, and SMM defined as a plasma cell disorder is now characterized by the presence of ≥ 3 g/dL serum M-protein and/or 10–60% bone marrow plasma cells (BMPCs), but with no evidence of myeloma-related symptomatology (hypercalcemia, renal insufficiency, anemia, or bone lesions (CRAB)) or any other myeloma-defining event (MDE) [2]. According to these recent update criteria, the definition of SMM excludes asymptomatic patients with BMPCs of 60% or more, serum free light chain (FLC) levels of ≥ 100, and those with two or more focal lesions in the skeleton as revealed by magnetic resonance imaging (MRI).

Kristinsson et al., based on the Swedish Myeloma Registry, has recently reported that 14% of patients diagnosed with myeloma had SMM, and, accordingly, the age-standardized incidence of SMM would be 0.44 cases per 100,000 people [3].

M.-V. Mateos (✉)
Hematology Department, Complejo Asistencial Universitario de Salamanca/Instituto Biosanitario de Salamanca (CAUSA/IBSAL), Paseo San Vicente, 58-182, 37007 Salamanca, Spain
e-mail: mvmateos@usal.es

J. San-Miguel
Clinica Universidad de Navarra, Pamplona, Spain

© Springer International Publishing AG 2018
S.Z. Usmani, A.K. Nooka (eds.), *Personalized Therapy for Multiple Myeloma*,
https://doi.org/10.1007/978-3-319-61872-2_1

Table 1.1 Differential diagnosis of MGUS, SMM, and symptomatic MM

Feature	MGUS	SMM	MM
Serum M-protein	<3 g/dL and	≥3 g/dL and/or	
Clonal BMPC infiltration	<10%	10–60%	≥10% or biopsy-proven plasmacytoma
Symptomatology	Absence of CRAB[a]	Absence of MDE[b] or amyloidosis	Presence of MDE[b]

[a]CRAB includes (1) hypercalcemia, serum calcium >0.25 mmol/L (>1 mg/dL) higher than the upper limit of normal or >2.75 mmol/L (>11 mg/dL); (2) renal insufficiency, serum creatinine >177 μmol/L (2 mg/dL) or creatinine clearance <40 mL/min; (3) anemia, hemoglobin value of >2 g/dL below the lower normal limit, or a hemoglobin value <10 g/dL; (4) bone lesions, one or more osteolytic lesion revealed by skeletal radiography, CT, or PET-CT
[b]MDE: Myeloma-defining events include CRAB symptoms (above) or any one or more of the following biomarkers of malignancy—clonal bone marrow plasma cell percentage ≥ 60%; involved/uninvolved serum free light chain ratio ≥ 100; >1 focal lesions revealed by MRI studies

1.2 Differential Diagnosis with Other Entities

SMM must be distinguished from other plasma cell disorders, such as monoclonal gammopathy of undetermined significance (MGUS) and symptomatic MM (Table 1.1). The MGUS entity is characterized by a level of serum M-protein of <3 g/dL plus <10% plasma cell infiltration in the bone marrow, with no CRAB and no MDE. Symptomatic MM must always have CRAB symptomatology or MDE, in conjunction with ≥10% clonal BMPC infiltration or biopsy-proven bony or extramedullary plasmacytoma [2].

End-organ damage often needs to be correctly evaluated to distinguish myeloma-related symptomatology from some signs or symptoms that could otherwise be attributed to comorbidities or concomitant diseases [4].

Due to the updated IMWG criteria for the diagnosis of MM, there are some specific assessments to which physicians have to pay attention in order to make a correct diagnosis of SMM [2].

1. For evaluation of bone disease, the IMWG recommends to perform in all patients with suspected SMM one of the following procedures: skeletal survey, ^{18}F-fluorodeoxyglucose (FDG) positron emission tomography (PET)/computed tomography (CT), or low-dose whole-body CT be carried out, with the exact modality determined by availability and resources. The aim is to exclude the presence of osteolytic bone lesions, currently defined by the presence of at least one lesion (≥5 mm) revealed by X-ray, CT, or PET-CT. In addition, whole-body MRI of the spine and pelvis is a mandatory component of the initial workup. It provides detailed information about not only bone marrow involvement but also the presence of focal lesions that predict more rapid progression to

symptomatic MM. Hillengass et al. reported in 2010 that the presence of more than one focal lesion in whole-body MRI was associated with a significantly shorter median time to progression (TTP) to active disease (13 months), as compared to patients without focal lesions [5]. Kastritis and colleagues reported similar results after the analysis of a subgroup of patients who underwent spinal MRI and were followed up for a minimum of 2.5 years. The median TTP to symptomatic disease was 14 months when more than one focal lesion was present [6]. Therefore, if more than one focal lesion in MRI is present in SMM patients, this entity should no longer be considered as SMM but as MM, according to the current IMWG criteria. It is important to emphasize that they should be unequivocal focal lesions of >5 mm.

2. With respect to bone marrow infiltration, the Mayo Clinic group evaluated BMPC infiltration in a cohort of 651 patients and found that 21 (3.2%) had an extreme infiltration ($\geq$ 60%) [7]. This group of patients had a median TTP to active disease of 7.7 months, with a 95% risk of progression at 2 years. This finding was subsequently validated in a study of 96 patients with SMM, in whom a median TTP of 15 months was reported for the group of patients with this extreme infiltration [8]. In a third study, 6 of 121 patients (5%) with SMM were found to have $\geq$60% BMPC, and all progressed to MM within 2 years [9]. Therefore, if $\geq$60% of clonal plasma cell infiltration is present either in bone marrow aspirate or biopsy, the diagnosis of SMM should be replaced by MM. Additional assessments, for example, by flow cytometry or by identifying cytogenetic abnormalities in SMM patients, are not mandatory but can help to estimate the risk of progression to active disease.

3. With respect to the serum free light chain (FLC) assay, Larsen et al. studied 586 patients with SMM to determine whether there was a threshold FLC ratio that predicted 85% of progression risk at 2 years. They found a serum involved/uninvolved FLC ratio of at least 100 in 15% of patients, and their risk of progression to symptomatic disease was 72% [10]. Similar results were obtained in a study by Kastritis and colleagues from the Greek Myeloma group. In their study of 96 SMM patients, 7% had an involved/uninvolved FLC ratio of $\geq$100 and almost all progressed within 18 months [8]. In a third study, the risk of progression within 2 years was 64% [9]. Therefore, physicians must perform the sFLC assay at the moment SMM is first suspected, and, if the involved/uninvolved ratio is $\geq$100, a diagnosis of active MM instead of SMM should be established.

If, after considering the specific assessments mentioned above (Table 1.2), a diagnosis of SMM is finally made, the serum and urine M-component, hemoglobin, calcium, and creatinine levels should be reevaluated 2–3 months later in order to confirm the stability of these parameters. The frequency of the subsequent follow-up exams should be adapted on the basis of risk factors for progression to symptomatic MM (see below).

Table 1.2 Workup for newly diagnosed SMM patients

• Medical history and physical examination
• Hemogram
• Biochemical studies, including of creatinine and calcium levels; Beta2-microglobulin, LDH and albumin

• Protein studies
  – Total serum protein and serum electrophoresis (serum M-protein)
  – 24-h urine sample protein electrophoresis (urine M-protein)
  – Serum and urine immunofixation
• Serum free light chain measurement (sFLC ratio)

• Bone marrow aspirate ± biopsy: infiltration by clonal plasma cells, flow cytometry, and fluorescence in situ hybridization analysis
• Skeletal survey, CT, or PET-CT
• MRI of thoracic and lumbar spine and pelvis; ideally, whole-body MRI

FLC free light chain, *CT* computed tomography, *PET-CT* ^{18}F-fluorodeoxyglucose (FDG) positron emission tomography (PET)/CT, *MRI* magnetic resonance imaging

1.3 Are There Risk Models Predicting the Progression Risk to MM?

The annual risk of progression from SMM to symptomatic MM is 10% per year for the first 5 years, 5% per year during the following 5 years, and only 1% per year after 10 years [11]. Though most patients diagnosed with SMM will progress to symptomatic MM and will need to start treatment, SMM is not a uniform disorder.

Several groups have reported possible predictors of progression to symptomatic MM, and this information could be useful for physicians and can help to explain to patients their risk of progression to active MM (Table 1.3).

1.3.1 Size of Serum M-Protein and the Extent of Marrow Involvement

Mayo Clinic group [11] proposed three SMM subgroups according to BMPC infiltration and the size of the serum M-protein. Group 1 was characterized by ≥3 g/dL of M-protein and ≥10% of plasma cells in bone marrow, with a median TTP to symptomatic MM of 2 years. Group 2 featured ≤3 g/dL of M-protein and ≥10% BMPC M-protein with a median TTP of 8 years. Group 3 had ≥3 g/dL of M-protein but <10% BMPC infiltration, resulting in a median TTP of 19 years.

1.3.2 Serum Free Light Chain Ratio

The Mayo Clinic group also evaluated the previously described patient population to identify the risk of progression to symptomatic MM on the basis of a free light chain (FLC) assay. A kappa/lambda FLC ratio between 0.125 and 8 was found to be

Table 1.3 Smoldering MM: markers predicting progression to symptomatic MM

Features for identifying high-risk SMM patients: 50% at 2 years

- *Tumor burden*
  - ≥10% clonal plasma cell bone marrow infiltration plus
  - ≥3 g/dL of serum M-protein and
  - Serum free light chain ratio between 0.125 and 8
  - Bence Jones proteinuria positive from 24-h urine sample
  - Peripheral blood circulating plasma cells >5 × 10⁶/L

- *Immunophenotyping characterization and immunoparesis*
  - ≥95% of aberrant plasma cells by flow within the plasma cell bone marrow compartment plus
  - immunoparesis (>25% decrease in one or both uninvolved immunoglobulins relative to the lowest normal value)

- *Cytogenetic abnormalities*
  - Presence of t(4;14)
  - Presence of del17p
  - Gains of 1q24
  - Hyperdiploidy
  - Gene expression profiling risk score > −0.26

- *Pattern of serum M-component evolution*
  - Evolving type: if M-protein ≥3 g/dL, increase of at least 10% within the first 6 months. If M-protein <3 g/dL, annual increase of M-protein for 3 years.
  - Increase in the M-protein to ≥3 g/dL over the 3 months since the previous determination

- *Imaging assessments*
  - MRI: radiological progressive disease (MRI-PD) was defined as newly detected focal lesions (FLs) or increase in diameter of existing FL and a novel or progressive diffuse infiltration
  - Positive PET/CT with no underlying osteolytic lesion

MRI magnetic resonance imaging, *PET-CT* ¹⁸F-fluorodeoxyglucose (FDG) positron emission tomography (PET)/CT

associated with an increase in the risk of progression to symptomatic MM. This parameter was added to their previous score, which considered the size of serum M-protein and BMPC infiltration, to refine the Mayo risk stratification model. This yielded three groups, with a median TTP of 1.9 years for the high-risk group, whose members exhibited all three defined risk factors [12].

The Danish Myeloma group did not find in the analysis of his registry any significant threshold for the serum free light chain ratio; therefore, they do not support the recent IMWG proposal that identifies patients with a FLC ratio above 100 as having ultra-high risk of transformation to MM [13].

1.3.3 Immunophenotyping and Immunoparesis

Multiparameter flow cytometry (MFC) to identify the immunophenotypic profile of plasma cells in SMM has been evaluated by the Spanish Myeloma group. We reported that the presence of an aberrant BMPC phenotype in the vast majority of PC (≥95% phenotypically abnormal plasma cells from total PC), determined by

MFC (defined as the overexpression of CD56 and CD19, CD45 negative, and/or decreased reactivity for CD38) was the most important predictor of early progression from SMM to active MM [14]. The presence of immunoparesis (i.e., a decrease in one or two of the uninvolved immunoglobulins to 25% below the lowest normal value) also emerged as a significant independent prognostic characteristic. Based on these two parameters, the Spanish group proposed a scoring system that stratify SMM patients into three categories with a median TTP of 23 months when the two risk factors were present, compared with 73 months when only one was present, and not reached when neither was present [15].

The Danish Myeloma registry has recently reported that both an M-protein ≥30 g/L and immunoparesis significantly influenced TTP (HR 2.7 95% CI(1.5;4.7) $p = 0.001$ and HR 3.3 95% CI(1.4;7.8) $p = 0.002$, respectively) to MM [13].

1.3.4 Peripheral Blood Circulating Plasma Cells

The Mayo Clinic group has also evaluated the role of peripheral blood circulating PCs in 171 SMM patients, and in those (15%) who had high levels of circulating PCs ($>5 \times 10^6$/L and/or $>5\%$ PCs per 100 cytoplasmic immunoglobulin (Ig)-positive mononuclear cells), the progression risk at 2 years was significantly higher than for patients with low levels of circulating PC (71% vs. 24%; $p = 0.001$) [16].

1.3.5 Pattern of Serum M-Component Evolution

The pattern of evolution of the monoclonal component during the course of the disease enabled to identify two types of SMM: evolving and non-evolving. Based on the analysis of 207 SMM patients, the evolving type was defined by the following criteria: (1) if the concentration of M-protein was ≥3 g/dL at baseline, the evolving type featured an increase in M-protein of at least 10% within the first 6 months following diagnosis; (2) if the concentration of M-protein was <3 g/dL at baseline, the evolving type featured a progressive increase in M-protein in each consecutive annual measurement over a 3-year period [17]. The evolving pattern was recognized in 25% of patients, and was associated with a probability of progression of 45% at 2 years, with a median TTP to active MM of 3 years, compared with 19 years for those with the non-evolving type [18]. The SWOG group also found that patients with an increase in the M component ≥3 g/dL over the 3 months since their previous determination had an associated risk of progression of approximately 50% at 2 years [19].

1.3.6 Bence Jones Proteinuria

One-hundred and forty-seven SMM patients were examined for the presence of Bence Jones proteinuria at diagnosis, and its effect on progression to symptomatic disease was assessed. The study showed that in SMM patients in which the M-protein was defined by a complete immunoglobulin, but who were also positive for Bence Jones proteinuria, regardless of the amount, the risk of progression to active disease was significantly higher than in Bence Jones proteinuria-negative patients (22 vs. 83 months; $p < 0.001$). In addition, when Bence Jones proteinuria in the 24-h urine sample exceeded 500 mg, the risk was even higher, with a median TTP of 7 months [20].

1.3.7 Novel Imaging Assessments

The novel imaging assessments have contributed to the updated criteria for the definition of MM and SMM, as has been previously mentioned. However, the new imaging assessments can also help to predict progression risk in SMM. The first studies with spinal MRI were done in asymptomatic MM patients, and the presence of a focal pattern was associated with a shorter TTP as compared to that of a diffuse or variegated pattern (median, 6 vs. 16 vs. 22 months). Hillengass et al. have recently evaluated the role of MRI during the follow-up of patients with SMM. Radiological progressive disease (MRI-PD), which they defined as the detection of new focal lesions or the increase in diameter of existing focal lesions, and a novel or progressive diffuse infiltration, was identified as a feature for classifying SMM patients at high risk of progression to symptomatic disease [21]. The role of PET/CT has also been evaluated in SMM. The Italian group has recently reported that approximately 10% of SMM patients from a series of 73 patients had a positive result with PET/CT with no underlying osteolytic lesion, and this predicted for high risk of progression to symptomatic disease (48% at 2 years compared with 32% for PET/CT-negative patients; $p = 0.007$) [22]. The Mayo Clinic group also identified a subgroup within a series of 132 SMM patients who showed a positive result with PET/CT in which the rate of progression to MM within 2 years was 56%, as compared to 28% among PET/CT-negative patients ($p = 0.001$). The rate of progression was even higher among patients on whom PET/CT was performed within 3 months of their diagnosis of SMM (74% vs. 27% in PET/CT-negative patients) [23].

1.3.8 Cytogenetic Abnormalities

The Mayo Clinic group analyzed the cytogenetic abnormalities in a series of 351 SMM patients and identified a high-risk subgroup of patients with t(4;14) and/or del(17p) with a significantly shorter median TTP (24 months) as compared to the intermediate-, standard-, and low-risk patient subgroups [24]. The high risk of progression of SMM to MM with t(4;14) may be related to the fact that this abnormality is associated with markedly high free light chain ratios. However, the mechanism by which a high free light chain ratio is associated with higher risk of progression is not clear and is only partly related to renal failure from cast nephropathy. Neben et al. have identified t(4;14), gain of 1q21, or hyperdiploidy as being independent prognostic factors for a shorter TTP. The median TTP for patients with del(17p13) was 2.7 years (vs. 4.9 years for those without the deletion; $p = 0.019$), 2.9 years for patients with t(4;14) (vs. 5.2 years for those without the deletion; $p = 0.021$), and 3.7 years for patients with +1q21 (vs. 5.3 years for those without the deletion; $p = 0.013$). In addition, hyperdiploidy was associated with a significantly shorter median TTP of 3.9 years (compared with 5.7 years for non-hyperdiploid patients; $p = 0.036$) [25].

Finally, the Southwest Oncology Group (SWOG) evaluated the gene expression profiling 40 (GEP40) model in a group of 105 SMM patients. A gene signature derived from four genes, at an optimal binary cut-point of 9.28, identified 14 patients (13%) with a 2-year progression risk of 85.7%. Conversely, a low four-gene score (< 9.28) combined with baseline monoclonal protein <3 g/dL and albumin ≥3.5 g/dL identified 61 patients with low-risk SMM with a 5.0% chance of progression at 2 years [26].

In summary, the diagnosis of SMM is associated with a variable risk of progression to active disease, and the presence of the aforementioned prognostic factors can discriminate subgroups of patients with respect to their degree of risk (Table 1.3).

1.4   Stratification and Management of SMM Patients

The first step in clinical practice is to identify the risk of progression to active disease for each newly diagnosed SMM patient. The key question is which risk model is better for evaluating the risk of progression to symptomatic disease for each individual SMM patient. Both the Mayo Clinic and Spanish models have been validated in a prospective trial. However, new risk models are emerging that incorporate novel clinical and biological features [9, 11, 13, 15, 17, 19, 25, 27, 28] (Table 1.4). The components of these models are not identical, and each patient's risk should probably be defined on the basis of all the available data rather than through the use of a restricted model (Table 1.3). These models identified their risk factors as independent variables in multivariate analysis, so some of the features evaluated in each risk model can overlap but not all of them have to be present in an SMM patient to be defined as high risk.

SMM patients should be classified as follows:

1. Patients at low risk of progression who are characterized by the absence of the aforementioned high-risk factors (using the validated Mayo or the Spanish risk models), with a probability of progression at 5 years of only 8%. The patients in this group behave similarly to MGUS-like patients and should be followed annually.
2. The second group includes patients at intermediate risk of progression, and they only display some of the aforementioned high-risk factors. These are probably the true SMM patients. They have a risk of progression at 5 years of 42%, and they must be followed up every 6 months (except during the first year that should be followed every 3–4 months in order to exclude an SMM evolving form).

Table 1.4 Risk models for the stratification of SMM

Risk model	Risk of progression to MM	
Mayo Clinic		**Median TTP**
– ≥10% clonal PCBM infiltration	1 risk factor	10 years
– ≥3 g/dL of serum M-protein	2 risk factors	5 years
– Serum FLC ratio between <0.125 or >8	3 risk factors	1.9 years
Spanish Myeloma		**Median TTP**
– ≥95% of aberrant PCs by MFC	No risk factor	NR
– Immunoparesis	1 risk factor	6 years
	2 risk factors	1.9 years
Heidelberg		**3-year TTP**
– Tumor mass using the Mayo model	T-mass low + CA low risk	15%
– t(4;14), del17p, or +1q	T-mass low + CA high risk	42%
	T-mass high + CA low risk	64%
	T-mass high + CA high risk	55%
SWOG		**2-year TTP**
– Serum M-protein ≥2 g/dL	No risk factor	30%
– Involved FLC > 25 mg/dL	1 risk factor	29%
– GEP risk score > −0.26	≥2 risk factors	71%
Penn		**2-year TTP**
– ≥40% clonal PCBM infiltration	No risk factor	16%
– sFLC ratio ≥ 50	1 risk factor	44%
– Albumin ≤3.5 mg/dL	≥2 risk factors	81%
Japanese		**2-year TTP**
– Beta 2-microglobulin ≥2.5 mg/L	2 risk factors	67.5%
– M-protein increment rate > 1 mg/dL/day		
Czech and Heidelberg		**2-year TTP**
– Immunoparesis	No risk factor	5.3%
– Serum M-protein ≥2.3 g/dL	1 risk factors	7.5%
– Involved/uninvolved sFLC >30	2 risk factors	44.8%
	3 risk factors	81.3%
Barcelona		**2-year TTP**
– Evolving pattern = 2 points	0 points	2.4%
– Serum M-protein ≥3 g/dL = 1 point	1 point	31%
– Immunoparesis = 1 point	2 points	52%
	3 points	80%
Danish		**3-year TTP**
– Serum M-protein ≥3 g/dL	No risk factor	5%
– Immunoparesis	1 risk factor	21%
	2 risk factors	50%

3. The third group includes high-risk patients classified on the basis of one of the risk models mentioned above. Half of them will progress during the 2 years following diagnosis. This group of patients needs a close follow-up every 2–3 months. As there is not any treatment approved yet for these high-risk SMM patients, the best approach should be to refer them to specialized centers in MM therapy and to include them in clinical trials to better understand their biology and to confirm the survival benefit of early treatment in this cohort [29].

The Spanish Myeloma group (GEM/Pethema) conducted a phase 3 randomized trial in 119 SMM patients at high risk of progression to active disease (according to the Mayo and/or Spanish criteria) that compared early treatment with lenalidomide plus dexamethasone as induction followed by lenalidomide alone as maintenance versus observation. The primary end point was TTP to symptomatic MM, and after a median follow-up of 40 months, the median TTP was significantly longer in patients in the early treatment group than in the observation arm (not reached vs. 21 months; hazard ratio, HR = 5.59; $p < 0.001$). Secondary end points included response, OS, and safety. The PR or better after induction was 82%, including 14% of cases of stringent complete response (sCR) plus CR, and after maintenance the sCR/CR rate increased to 26%. The safety profile was acceptable and most of the adverse events reported were grade 1 or 2. The OS analysis showed that the 3-year survival rate was also higher for the group of patients who received early treatment with lenalidomide-based therapy (94% vs. 80%; HR = 3.24; $p = 0.03$) [30]. This study showed for the first time the potential for changing the treatment paradigm for high-risk SMM patients based on the efficacy of early treatment in terms of TTP to active disease and of OS. Moreover, several trials currently underway are currently investigating the role, on high-risk SMM patients, of novel agents such as lenalidomide alone, siltuximab (anti-IL6 monoclonal antibody), elotuzumab (anti-SLAMF7 monoclonal antibody), or lenalidomide-dexamethasone plus elotuzumab. Promising efficacy results have been reported for the combination of lenalidomide plus dexamethasone with the novel proteasome inhibitor carfilzomib in a series of 12 high-risk SMM patients. All patients achieved CR and most were in immunophenotypic CR [31]. The next step will be to develop a more intensive therapeutic approach for young high-risk SMM patients, similar to the treatment planned for young symptomatic MM patients, for whom "cure" should be the objective.

1.5 Conclusion and Future Directions

The treatment philosophy for MM patients has mainly focused on symptomatic patients. This approach is clearly different from those adopted to treat other malignancies, such as breast, colon, or prostate cancer, for which early intervention is not only appropriate but also essential for success and cure. This difference in philosophy arose for several reasons: (1) in the past, only a few drugs, most of which were alkylating agents, were available to treat MM; (2) the trials conducted in asymptomatic MM patients failed to produce a significant benefit; and (3) the risk of progression to active disease in SMM patients is relatively low (10% per year).

However, significant advances are being made in the understanding and management of SMM patients. From the biological point of view, different subgroups of SMM patients have been identified, including those patients with >60% PC or FLC ratio > 100 or two or more focal lesions, that are now considered as active MM patients in which treatment should be started before myeloma-related symptoms develop.

We will soon have the results from several current trials conducted in high-risk SMM patients, which will enable us to offer early treatment for a selected group of asymptomatic MM patients with the confidence that some of them will be "cured." The cure-versus-control debate is particularly pertinent in asymptomatic myeloma patients. Some physicians argue in favor of controlling the disease through continuous oral therapy mainly based on immunomodulatory agents, while others support the intensive therapy approaches, including high-dose therapy and transplant, with the objective of eradicating the disease.

Ongoing biological studies will also help us to better understand the pathogenesis of the disease and to identify the key drivers of the transition from monoclonal gammopathy to smoldering and symptomatic disease. These drivers may represent optimal targets for new therapeutic approaches.

References

1. Kyle RA, Greipp PR. Smoldering multiple myeloma. N Engl J Med. 1980;302(24):1347–9. doi:10.1056/NEJM198006123022405.
2. Rajkumar SV, Dimopoulos MA, Palumbo A, Blade J, Merlini G, Mateos MV, Kumar S, Hillengass J, Kastritis E, Richardson P, Landgren O, Paiva B, Dispenzieri A, Weiss B, LeLeu X, Zweegman S, Lonial S, Rosinol L, Zamagni E, Jagannath S, Sezer O, Kristinsson SY, Caers J, Usmani SZ, Lahuerta JJ, Johnsen HE, Beksac M, Cavo M, Goldschmidt H, Terpos E, Kyle RA, Anderson KC, Durie BG, Miguel JF. International Myeloma Working Group updated criteria for the diagnosis of multiple myeloma. Lancet Oncol. 2014b;15(12):e538–48. doi:10.1016/s1470-2045(14)70442-5.
3. Kristinsson SY, Holmberg E, Blimark C. Treatment for high-risk smoldering myeloma. N Engl J Med. 2013;369(18):1762–3. doi:10.1056/NEJMc1310911#SA1.
4. Blade J, Dimopoulos M, Rosinol L, Rajkumar SV, Kyle RA. Smoldering (asymptomatic) multiple myeloma: current diagnostic criteria, new predictors of outcome, and follow-up recommendations. J Clin Oncol. 2010;28(4):690–7. doi:10.1200/JCO.2009.22.2257.
5. Hillengass J, Fechtner K, Weber MA, Bauerle T, Ayyaz S, Heiss C, Hielscher T, Moehler TM, Egerer G, Neben K, Ho AD, Kauczor HU, Delorme S, Goldschmidt H. Prognostic significance of focal lesions in whole-body magnetic resonance imaging in patients with asymptomatic multiple myeloma. J Clin Oncol. 2010;28(9):1606–10. doi:10.1200/JCO.2009.25.5356.
6. Kastritis E, Moulopoulos LA, Terpos E, Koutoulidis V, Dimopoulos MA. The prognostic importance of the presence of more than one focal lesion in spine MRI of patients with asymptomatic (smoldering) multiple myeloma. Leukemia. 2014;28(12):2402–3. doi:10.1038/leu.2014.230.
7. Rajkumar SV, Larson D, Kyle RA. Diagnosis of smoldering multiple myeloma. N Engl J Med. 2011;365(5):474–5. doi:10.1056/NEJMc1106428.

8. Kastritis E, Terpos E, Moulopoulos L, Spyropoulou-Vlachou M, Kanellias N, Eleftherakis-Papaiakovou E, Gkotzamanidou M, Migkou M, Gavriatopoulou M, Roussou M, Tasidou A, Dimopoulos MA. Extensive bone marrow infiltration and abnormal free light chain ratio identifies patients with asymptomatic myeloma at high risk for progression to symptomatic disease. Leukemia. 2012;27(4):947–53.

9. Waxman AJ, Mick R, Garfall AL, Cohen A, Vogl DT, Stadtmauer EA, Weiss BM. Classifying ultra-high risk smoldering myeloma. Leukemia. 2014. doi:10.1038/leu.2014.313.

10. Larsen JT, Kumar SK, Dispenzieri A, Kyle RA, Katzmann JA, Rajkumar SV. Serum free light chain ratio as a biomarker for high-risk smoldering multiple myeloma. Leukemia. 2013;27(4):941–6. doi:10.1038/leu.2012.296.

11. Kyle RA, Remstein ED, Therneau TM, Dispenzieri A, Kurtin PJ, Hodnefield JM, Larson DR, Plevak MF, Jelinek DF, Fonseca R, Melton LJ 3rd, Rajkumar SV. Clinical course and prognosis of smoldering (asymptomatic) multiple myeloma. N Engl J Med. 2007;356(25):2582–90. doi:10.1056/NEJMoa070389.

12. Dispenzieri A, Kyle RA, Katzmann JA, Therneau TM, Larson D, Benson J, Clark RJ, Melton LJ 3rd, Gertz MA, Kumar SK, Fonseca R, Jelinek DF, Rajkumar SV. Immunoglobulin free light chain ratio is an independent risk factor for progression of smoldering (asymptomatic) multiple myeloma. Blood. 2008;111(2):785–9. doi:10.1182/blood-2007-08-108357.

13. Sorrig R, Klausen TW, Salomo M, Vangsted AJ, Ostergaard B, Gregersen H, Frolund UC, Andersen NF, Helleberg C, Andersen KT, Pedersen RS, Pedersen P, Abildgaard N, Gimsing P. Smoldering multiple myeloma risk factors for progression: a Danish population-based cohort study. Eur J Haematol. 2015. doi:10.1111/ejh.12728.

14. Perez-Persona E, Vidriales MB, Mateo G, Garcia-Sanz R, Mateos MV, de Coca AG, Galende J, Martin-Nunez G, Alonso JM, de Las HN, Hernandez JM, Martin A, Lopez-Berges C, Orfao A, San Miguel JF. New criteria to identify risk of progression in monoclonal gammopathy of uncertain significance and smoldering multiple myeloma based on multiparameter flow cytometry analysis of bone marrow plasma cells. Blood. 2007;110(7):2586–92.

15. Perez-Persona E, Mateo G, Garcia-Sanz R, Mateos MV, de Las HN, de Coca AG, Hernandez JM, Galende J, Martin-Nunez G, Barez A, Alonso JM, Martin A, Lopez-Berges C, Orfao A, San Miguel JF, Vidriales MB. Risk of progression in smouldering myeloma and monoclonal gammopathies of unknown significance: comparative analysis of the evolution of monoclonal component and multiparameter flow cytometry of bone marrow plasma cells. Br J Haematol. 2010;148(1):110–4. doi:10.1111/j.1365-2141.2009.07929.x.

16. Bianchi G, Kyle RA, Larson DR, Witzig TE, Kumar S, Dispenzieri A, Morice WG, Rajkumar SV. High levels of peripheral blood circulating plasma cells as a specific risk factor for progression of smoldering multiple myeloma. Leukemia. 2013;27(3):680–5. doi:10.1038/leu.2012.237.

17. Fernández de Larrea C, Isola I, Cibeira MT, Rosiñol L, Calvo X, Tovar N, Elena M, Magnano L, Aróstegui JI, Rozman M, Yagüe J, Bladé J. Smoldering multiple myeloma: impact of the evolving pattern on early progression. Blood. 2014;124(21):3363–3.

18. Rosinol L, Blade J, Esteve J, Aymerich M, Rozman M, Montoto S, Gine E, Nadal E, Filella X, Queralt R, Carrio A, Montserrat E. Smoldering multiple myeloma: natural history and recognition of an evolving type. Br J Haematol. 2003;123(4):631–6.

19. Dhodapkar MV, Sexton R, Waheed S, Usmani S, Papanikolaou X, Nair B, Petty N, Shaughnessy JD Jr, Hoering A, Crowley J, Orlowski RZ, Barlogie B. Clinical, genomic, and imaging predictors of myeloma progression from asymptomatic monoclonal gammopathies (SWOG S0120). Blood. 2014;123(1):78–85. doi:10.1182/blood-2013-07-515239.

20. Gonzalez de la Calle V, Garcia-Sanz R, Sobejano E, Ocio EM, Puig N, Gutierrez NC, Melón A, Gonzalez J, Garcia de Coca A, Hernandez JM, Hernandez R, Barez A, Alonso JM, Aguilera C, Escalante F, Martin G, Lopez R, de la Fuente P, Mateos M-V. Bence Jones proteinuria in smoldering multiple myeloma as predictor marker of progression to symptomatic multiple myeloma. Blood. 2014;124(21):3369–9.

21. Merz M, Hielscher T, Wagner B, Sauer S, Shah S, Raab MS, Jauch A, Neben K, Hose D, Egerer G, Weber MA, Delorme S, Goldschmidt H, Hillengass J. Predictive value of longitudi-

nal whole-body magnetic resonance imaging in patients with smoldering multiple myeloma. Leukemia. 2014. doi:10.1038/leu.2014.75.

22. Zamagni E, Nanni C, Gay F, Pezzi A, Patriarca F, Bello M, Rambaldi I, Tacchetti P, Hillengass J, Gamberi B, Pantani L, Magarotto V, Versari A, Offidani M, Zannetti B, Carobolante F, Balma M, Musto P, Rensi M, Mancuso K, Dimitrakopoulou-Strauss A, Chauvie S, Rocchi S, Fard N, Marzocchi G, Storto G, Ghedini P, Palumbo A, Fanti S, Cavo M. 18F-FDG PET/CT focal, but not osteolytic, lesions predict the progression of smoldering myeloma to active disease. Leukemia. 2016;30(2):417–22. doi:10.1038/leu.2015.291.

23. Siontis B, Kumar S, Dispenzieri A, Drake MT, Lacy MQ, Buadi F, Dingli D, Kapoor P, Gonsalves W, Gertz MA, Rajkumar SV. Positron emission tomography-computed tomography in the diagnostic evaluation of smoldering multiple myeloma: identification of patients needing therapy. Blood cancer journal. 2015;5:e364. doi:10.1038/bcj.2015.87.

24. Rajkumar SV, Gupta V, Fonseca R, Dispenzieri A, Gonsalves WI, Larson D, Ketterling RP, Lust JA, Kyle RA, Kumar SK. Impact of primary molecular cytogenetic abnormalities and risk of progression in smoldering multiple myeloma. Leukemia. 2013. doi:10.1038/leu.2013.86.

25. Neben K, Jauch A, Hielscher T, Hillengass J, Lehners N, Seckinger A, Granzow M, Raab MS, Ho AD, Goldschmidt H, Hose D. Progression in smoldering myeloma is independently determined by the chromosomal abnormalities del(17p), t(4;14), gain 1q, hyperdiploidy, and tumor load. J Clin Oncol. 2013;31(34):4325–32. doi:10.1200/jco.2012.48.4923.

26. Khan R, Dhodapkar M, Rosenthal A, Heuck C, Papanikolaou X, Qu P, van Rhee F, Zangari M, Jethava Y, Epstein J, Yaccoby S, Hoering A, Crowley J, Petty N, Bailey C, Morgan G, Barlogie B. Four genes predict high risk of progression from smoldering to symptomatic multiple myeloma (SWOG S0120). Haematologica. 2015;100(9):1214–21. doi:10.3324/haematol.2015.124651.

27. Hajek R, Sandecka V, Seckinger A, Spicka I, Scudla V, Gregora E, Radocha J, Brozova L, Jarkovsky J, Rihova L, Mikulasova A, Starostka D, Walterova L, Adamova D, Kessler P, Brejcha M, Vonke I, Obernauerova J, Valentova K, Adam Z, Minarik J, Straub J, Gumulec J, Ho AD, Hillengass J, Goldschmidt H, Maisnar V, Hose D. Prediction of progression of smouldering into therapy requiring multiple myeloma by easily accessible clinical factors [in 527 patients]. Blood. 2014;124(21):2071–1.

28. Muta T, Iida S, Matsue K, Sunami K, Isoda J, Harada N, Saburi Y, Okamura S, Kumagae K, Watanabe J, Kuroda J, Aoki K, Ogawa R, Miyamoto T, Akashi K, Takamatsu Y. Predictive significance of serum beta 2-microglobulin levels and M-protein velocity for symptomatic progression of smoldering multiple myeloma. Blood. 2014;124(21):3379–9.

29. Mateos MV, San Miguel JF. New approaches to smoldering myeloma. Curr Hematol Malig Rep. 2013. doi:10.1007/s11899-013-0174-1.

30. Mateos MV, Hernandez MT, Giraldo P, de la Rubia J, de Arriba F, Lopez Corral L, Rosinol L, Paiva B, Palomera L, Bargay J, Oriol A, Prosper F, Lopez J, Olavarria E, Quintana N, Garcia JL, Blade J, Lahuerta JJ, San Miguel JF. Lenalidomide plus dexamethasone for high-risk smoldering multiple myeloma. N Engl J Med. 2013;369(5):438–47. doi:10.1056/NEJMoa1300439.

31. Landgren O, Roschewski M, Mailankody S, Kwok M, Manasanch EE, Bhutani M, Tageja N, Kazandjian D, Zingone A, Costello R, Burton D, Zhang Y, Wu P, Carter G, Mulquin M, Zuchlinski D, Carpenter A, Gounden V, Morrison C, Maric I, Calvo KR, Braylan RC, Yuan C, Stetler-Stevenson M, Arthur DC, Lindenberg L, Karen K, Choyke P, Steinberg SM, Figg WD, Korde N. Carfilzomib, lenalidomide, and dexamethasone in high-risk smoldering multiple myeloma: final results from the NCI phase 2 pilot study. Blood. 2014;124(21):4746–6.

Risk Stratification in Newly Diagnosed Transplant-Eligible Multiple Myeloma

Megan H. Jagosky, Alankrita Taneja, and Manisha Bhutani

2.1   Introduction

Complex interplay between biology, chromosomal abnormalities, gene expression profiles (GEP), and staging affects prognostication of multiple myeloma (MM). With novel therapies being developed, it is increasingly important to risk stratify the affected population by using available prognostic markers. Risk stratification is not unique to MM. Like other hematologic malignancies, the ability to predict outcome based on risk group is important when counseling the patient regarding the therapeutic outcomes and risk/benefit of treatment. The risk classification schema for MM has evolved over the years in parallel with changing treatment landscape and diagnostic approaches. Most of the risk factors are derived from data on patients treated in the era before novel agents. The traditional prognostic markers continue to be relevant and in the modern era these are used to investigate how novel agents can influence the patient's risk. The International Myeloma Working Group (IMWG) panel provided its updated recommendations for risk stratification in 2014 [1]. According to IMWG, the high-risk patients are distinguished as having a median overall survival (OS) of 2 years or less despite best therapies and low-risk patients as those who could potentially survive more than 10 years with treatment. Autologous stem cell transplant (ASCT) continues to hold its place for all eligible patients in an era when patients have multiple regimen options for induction, consolidation, and maintenance therapy. Integrating novel prognostic factors and updating risk classification schema within the context of emerging therapeutic paradigms is an area of flux. With increasing treatment choices and improved outcomes, risk

M.H. Jagosky • A. Taneja • M. Bhutani, M.D. (✉)
Department of Hematologic Oncology, Blood Disorders and Bone Marrow Transplantation,
Levine Cancer Institute, Carolinas HealthCare System,
1021 Morehead Medical Drive, Suite 5300, Charlotte, NC 28204, USA
e-mail: manisha.bhutani@carolinashealthcare.org

© Springer International Publishing AG 2018
S.Z. Usmani, A.K. Nooka (eds.), *Personalized Therapy for Multiple Myeloma*,
https://doi.org/10.1007/978-3-319-61872-2_2

stratification assumes more importance as fine-tuned therapeutic plans can be developed for different risk groups.

2.2   Why Is Risk Stratification Important?

Risk classification is frequently used by physicians for counseling their patients regarding life expectancy, disease control, health-related quality of life, and treatment complications while weighing the cost and benefit of different therapeutic options. Unlike acute leukemia and Hodgkin lymphoma, MM has little randomized data on benefit of altering treatment for high-risk group or for de-escalating treatment for the low-risk group. Nonetheless, risk grouping provides a useful framework for rational selection taking into consideration the cost of drugs, toxicities, and efficacies. For high-risk disease, physicians and patients may be more inclined to use potent treatments with potentially greater toxicity and expense, whereas for low-risk disease, less toxic and more affordable regimens may be preferred even with a slight compromise in efficacy. These practices may vary according to the divergent viewpoint of cure (choosing a more aggressive approach) vs. control (choosing a less aggressive approach with focus on quality of life). Within the realm of clinical trials, risk stratification is used to define a class of patients to be included or excluded from studies that are designed for a specific risk group. Importantly, risk grouping creates a common nomenclature to allow patients, physicians, institutions, government agencies, and cooperative groups to present and/or compare outcome data in a uniform manner.

2.3   What Markers Determine the Risk?

Several markers reflecting biology, stage, disease burden, host characteristics, and response to therapy have been identified (Table 2.1) that predict outcome in MM. Most of these biomarkers are prognostic, which means they provide information about the outcome at the time of diagnosis or at various times during the recurrent disease, independent of therapy. In contrast, we have few predictive markers, which can provide information on the likelihood of response to a given therapeutic modality. For example, cereblon expression may predict resistance to immunomodulatory drug (IMiD) but by itself is not a prognostic factor [2]. Importantly, prognostic factors define the effects on the patient outcome and are useful in risk stratification, whereas predictive factors define the effect of treatment on the tumor.

Studies conducted in the 1960s and early 1970s identified a number of clinical and laboratory parameters that were proposed for staging myeloma burden [3, 4]. In 1975, Durie/Salmon (DS) myeloma staging system came to light. This system reflects disease burden based on the level and type of monoclonal protein, hemoglobin, calcium, and number of bone lesions [5]. Patients in each of the three stages are defined lower risk vs. higher risk based on creatinine level (substage A: serum creatinine <2 mg/dL; substage B: serum creatinine ≥2 mg/day). In the 1980s, serum

Table 2.1 Determinants of risk

Myeloma cell burden	Patient characteristics	Disease biology	Response to treatment
DS staging system	Age	LDH >300 IU/L	CR
ISS	Performance status, frailty	Plasma cell labeling ≥ 1%	Immunophenotypic CR
	Organ function	Conventional cytogenetics	Molecular CR
MRI (≥7 lesions, diffuse bone marrow involvement) FDG-PET (≥3 lesions, SUV >4.2, presence of extramedullary disease)	Comorbidity burden index	Interphase FISH – CD138 selection – Immunofluorescence of cytoplasmic Ig FISH	PET/MRI CR or resolution of lesions
Extramedullary disease	Geriatric assessment score	Gene expression profiling	
Plasma cell leukemia	Psychosocial profile		

DS Durie-Salmon, *ISS* International Staging System, *MRI* magnetic resonance imaging, *FDG-PET* fluorodeoxyglucose-positron emission tomography, *SUV* standardized uptake value, *LDH* lactate dehydrogenase, *FISH* fluorescence in situ hybridization, *Ig* immunoglobulin, *CR* complete response

β2-microglobulin became known as a reliable predictor of survival duration [6, 7]. In mid-1980s prognostic relevance of conventional cytogenetics by metaphase G-banding was described [8]. Subsequently, chromosomal abnormalities identified by interphase fluorescent in situ hybridization (FISH) were adapted as the key elements for defining risk categories [9]. The three-tier risk stratification system that we commonly use to classify newly diagnosed MM into standard, intermediate, and high risk of relapse is primarily based on the chromosomal abnormalities. Standard-risk disease is characterized by the absence of del(17p), t(4;14)(p16;q32), t(14;16) (q32;q23), or 1q21 amplification (1q21+) and is associated with a median OS of 50.5 months [10]. In contrast, high-risk disease is characterized by the presence of at least one of the previously mentioned abnormalities and is associated with a median OS of 24.5 months ($P < 0.001$) [10]. Patients harboring chromosomal aberrations, such as del(13), t(11;14), t(6;14), or hyperdiploidy in the absence of other high-risk defining features, generally have standard or intermediate-risk disease (Table 2.2).

In 2005, the International Staging System (ISS) was devised and quickly superseded the DS system. ISS is based on two simple inexpensive routine laboratory tests that reflect not just the tumor burden and renal function (β2-microglobulin) but also biologic impact of host-tumor interaction (albumin) [11]. The median OS of ISS stage III patients (serum β2-microglobulin >5.5 mg/mL) was reported as 29 months compared with patients classified as stage I myeloma (serum albumin

Table 2.2 Risk classification based on FISH and conventional cytogenetics

Category	Genes/ chromosomes	Frequency (%)	Risk	Comments
Hyperdiploidy	Usually trisomies involving odd-numbered chromosomes except for chromosome 1,13, and 21	42	Standard	Hyperdiploidy is an initiating pathogenetic event
Monosomy 13 or del(13q), in the absence of other high-risk abnormalities		15 (metaphase karyotype) 50 (FISH)	Standard	The historically negative impact has been related to overlap with t(4;14) and/or del17p
Ig H translocated		40		
t(11;14) (q13; q32)	*CCND1* (cyclin D1)	15–20	Standard or intermediate	
t(4;14) (p16; q32)	*FGFR-3* and MMSET	12–15	High	
t(14;16) (q32; q23)	*C-MAF*	3	High	
t(14;20) (q32; q11)	*MAFB*	1	High	
t(6;14) (p21; q32) and other	*CCND3* (cyclin D3)	<5	Standard	
Combined hyperdiploidy + high-risk cytogenetics		15	Undetermined	It is unclear if the favorable prognostic impact of hyperdiploidy is lost in such cases
Isolated Monosomy 14, lack both IgH translocations and trisomies	Few cases may represent 14q32 translocations involving unknown partner chromosomes	4.5	Undetermined	
Other cytogenetic abnormalities in absence of IgH translocations or trisomy or monosomy 14		5.5	Undetermined	
Normal		3	Standard	

Table 2.2 (continued)

Category	Genes/ chromosomes	Frequency (%)	Risk	Comments
1p deletions	*CDKN2C*, *FAF1*. *FAM46C*	11–30	High	Deletion of 1p32.3 and 1p12 has been associated with impaired OS in myeloma patients receiving ASCT
Gain 1 q21	*CKS1B*, *PMSD4*	40	High	Patients with ≥3 copies of 1q have a worse treatment outcome The data is conflicting about 1q21+. Some reports have shown 1q21+ to be an independent prognostic factor [61], whereas others have not [63]. Although its role as a poor prognostic factor is controversial, the lack of 1q21+ is useful in identifying patients with standard prognosis [64]
Del 17p	The molecular target of del(17p) may be *TP53*	7	High	These patients present with more aggressive disease, extramedullary disease, and central nervous system involvement At present, it is not clear what minimum percentage of cells carrying del(17p) is required to confer adverse prognosis. Minimal percentages of 20% and 60% have been recommended

≥3.5 mg/mL, serum β2-microglobulin <3.5 mg/mL), who had a median OS of 62 months. The strength of the ISS is that it is a robust staging system that has been validated and is applicable across geographical areas. It maintains prognostic efficacy in a variety of clinical situations, namely, older (>65 years) vs. younger patients and treatment with conventional vs. ASCT. The main drawback, however, is that the FISH/cytogenetic features were not included in the derivation of ISS.

In addition to markers used in DS and ISS staging system, high serum lactate dehydrogenase (LDH), an indicator of rapid tumor turnover, is another marker of inferior outcome. It has consistently been associated with short OS in studies conducted before and in the era of novel agents [12, 13]. Within each ISS group, the presence of high LDH is associated with a worse median OS.

GEP signature is also an important tool that provides supplementary information regarding prognosis. The first comprehensive GEP signature of newly diagnosed MM patients was published by the Arkansas group in 2002 [14]. Thereafter, numerous GEP signatures have been identified in the context of retrospective and prospective analyses for both newly diagnosed and relapsed patient populations. Examples include UAMS 70-gene signature [15], EMC 92-gene signature [16], 17-gene signature by UAMS [15], 15-gene signature in the IFM trials [17], and a 6-gene signature in the MRC Myeloma IX trial [18]. GEP signatures are particularly effective in identifying high-risk group comprising 15% of new cases of MM with very poor outcomes. The technology of GEP is robust with good interlaboratory agreement. Unfortunately, widespread adoption of GEP in the clinics has been hindered by concern over variation between published signatures, difficulty in physician interpretation, and the challenge of obtaining sufficient genetic material from limited patient specimens. The IMWG conducted a study to unify the GEP signatures using prognostic modeling and found that the combination of prognostic signatures is generally better than single signature [19]. In this study, the simple average of EMC 92 and HZDC2 indices performed the best across datasets that comprised newly diagnosed and relapsed patients treated with novel agents and ASCT. Beyond lower-resolution genetic analyses like cytogenetics and FISH, clonal and subclonal heterogeneity in MM has been comprehensively characterized by genome-based diagnostic approaches including whole exome sequencing and whole genome sequencing (WGS). Other newer approaches to predict survival include analysis of microRNAs, custom capture mutation analysis, and evaluation of methylation and splicing patterns.

2.4   What Is the Value of Combined Prognostic Models?

Because individual prognostic factors do not capture the full heterogeneity in outcome, several studies have used models combined models combining ISS with FISH cytogenetics and other prognostic features (Table 2.3). These combined models more accurately segregate patients into risk groups that better predict outcome for transplanted MM patients. Integrated prognostic models have shown to outperform prediction based on conventional clinical and cytogenetic factors alone.

Table 2.3 Staging systems and risk classification systems for newly diagnosed multiple myeloma

Classification	Stage	Frequency (%)	OS
DS [5] (substage A: serum creatinine <2 mg/dL; and substage B: serum creatinine ≥2 mg/day)	I All the following: Hb > 10 g/dL Ca ≤ 12 mg/dL Normal or solitary plasmacytoma on skeletal survey Serum M protein <50 g/L for IgG; <3 g/dL for IgA; Bence Jones protein <4 g/24 h	7.5 (IA) 0.5 (IB)	50% at 62 months 50% at 22 months
	II Neither stage I nor stage III	22 (IIA) 4 (IIB)	50% at 58 months 50% at 34 months
	III One of the following: Hb < 8.5 g/dL Ca > 12 mg/dL Advanced lytic bone lesions (scale 3) Serum M protein >7 g/dL for IgG; >5 g/dL for IgA; Bence Jones protein >12 g/24 h	49 (IIIA) 17 (IIIB)	50% at 45 months 50% at 24 months
ISS [11]	I Serum β2-microglobulin <3.5 mg/L, serum albumin ≥3.5 g/dL	30	50% at 62 months
	II Not fitting to stage I or II	37.5	50% at 44 months
	III Serum β2-microglobulin ≥5.5 mg/L	34	50% at 29 months
mSMART (http://www.msmart.org)	Standard All other cytogenetics including trisomies (hyperdiploidy), t(11;14), t(6;14)	NA	NA
	Intermediate t(4;14) 1q gain High PC-S phase	NA	NA
	High del (17p13) t(14;16) t(14;20) LDH ≥2 times institutional upper limit of normal Features of primary plasma cell leukemia High-risk gene expression profiling signature	NA	NA

(continued)

Table 2.3 (continued)

Classification	Stage	Frequency (%)	OS
ISS + Cytogenetic abnormalities in ASCT-eligible [60]	Favorable ISS stage I and not (4;14) or del(17p13)	42	72% at 60 months
	Intermediate Neither favorable nor poor	44	62% at 60 months
	Poor ISS stage II/III and t(4;14) or del(17p13)	14	41% at 60 months
ISS + Cytogenetic abnormalities in ASCT eligible and ineligible patients with NDMM [61]	Favorable ISS stage I/II and no t(4;14), t(14;16), +1q21, del(13), del(17) or ISS stage I with 1 CA	38	50% at 68 months
	Intermediate ISS stage I and >1 CA, or ISS stage II/III and 1 CA, or ISS III and no CA	48	50% at 41 months
	Ultra-high ISS II/III with >1 CA	14	50% at 19 months
ISS + CA in ASCT eligible and ineligible patients with NDMM [62]	Favorable ISS I/II and no t(4;14) or del(17p13)	51	77% at 48 months
	Intermediate ISS III and no t(4;14) or del(17p13) or ISS I and t(4;14) or del(17p13)	29	45% at 48 months
	Poor ISS II/II and t(4;14) or del(17p13)	20	33% at 48 months
ISS + CA + LDH in ASCT-eligible patients with NDMM [21]	Score 0 No adverse factors of the other categories	47–63	93% at 24 months
	Score 1 Only one adverse factor of categories 2 and 3	28–34	85% at 24 months
	Score 2 High LDH, ISS III, no t(4;14) or del(17p13)	2–5	67% at 24 months
	Score 3 t(4;14) and/or del(17p13), and ISS III, and/or high LDH	5–13	55% at 24 months

Table 2.3 (continued)

Classification	Stage	Frequency (%)	OS
Revised ISS in ASCT-eligible and ASCT-ineligible with NDMM [20]	Stage I • Serum albumin ≥3.5 gm/dL • Serum beta-2-microglobulin <3.5 mg/L • No high-risk cytogenetics • Normal serum LDH	28	82% at 46 months
	Stage II Not fitting stage I or III	62	62% at 46 months
	Stage III • Serum beta-2-microglobulin >5.5 mg/L • High-risk cytogenetics [t(4;14), t(14;16), or del(17p)] or elevated serum LDH	10	40% at 46 months
GEP signatures	UAMS 70-gene [15]		
	High risk	13	28% at 60 months
	Low risk		78% at 60 months
	IFM 15-gene [17]		
	High risk	25	47% at 36 months
	Low risk		90% at 36 months
	EMC 92-gene [16]		
	High risk (validation set of MRC IX- transplant eligible)	20	50% at 40 months
	Low risk		50% at 62 months

DS Durie and Salmon, *ISS* International Staging System, *NDMM* Newly diagnosed multiple myeloma, *CA* cytogenetic abnormality, *LDH* lactate dehydrogenase, *GEP* gene expression profiling, *ASCT* autologous stem cell transplant, *mSMART* Mayo Stratification of Myeloma and Risk-Adapted Therapy, *Hb* hemoglobin, *Ca* calcium, *UAMS* University of Arkansas for Medical Sciences, *IFM* Intergroupe Francophone du Myélome, *NA* not available, *OS* overall survival

IMWG published revised ISS (R-ISS) in 2015 that incorporates the original ISS, cytogenetic abnormalities, and serum LDH [20]. R-ISS provides a comprehensive and practical risk stratification of newly diagnosed MM, including both young and elderly patients, that allows a clear identification of three stages with different survival durations. R-ISS stage I includes ISS stage I, no high-risk cytogenetic abnormalities, and normal LDH; R-ISS stage III includes ISS stage III with high-risk cytogenetic abnormalities and/or high LDH levels; and R-ISS stage II includes all the remaining. High-risk cytogenetic abnormalities included del(17p), t(4;14), and/or t(4;16), whereas all other cytogenetic/FISH markers were considered standard risk. Patients with R-ISS stage I, II, and III had 5-year OS rates of 82%, 62%, and 40%, respectively. Another study that combined ISS, cytogenetic abnormalities, and LDH defined four risk categories: in the very low-risk category, the 2-year OS was 93%. In contrast, the 2-year OS was 55% in the very high-risk category [21]. ISS has also been combined with GEP classifiers. By combining the EMC 92-gene classifier with ISS, patients were effectively stratified into four risk groups, including a distinctive low-risk group of 38% and a high-risk group of 17% [19]. In summary, combined risk models including ISS and genetic risk stratification robustly characterize those patients who have a high risk of early death from progression within the first 2 years of MM diagnosis.

2.5   Does Depth of Treatment Response Affect Risk Stratification?

Although pretreatment disease characteristics remain the hallmark of prognostication, posttreatment parameters such as minimal residual disease (MRD) assessment and degree of response to therapy possess the ability to further refine the prognosis. Not only does response to treatment provide a synopsis of therapeutic resistance, it also helps determine the impact of dosage, compliance, and other unknown biology factors influencing the effectiveness of treatment. The proportion of patients achieving CR has increased through the introduction of novel agents and use of ASCT, necessitating more stringent definitions for assessing the exact magnitude of response in MM. The IMWG revised the reporting criteria, adding immunophenotypic CR and molecular CR categories [22]. Thus, more sensitive approaches like multiparameter flow cytometry (MFC) and molecular techniques like allele-specific oligonucleotide polymerase chain reaction (ASO-PCR) and NGS are being adapted for response and MRD assessment. More than a decade ago, Rawstron et al. first identified MRD as an independent predictor of relapse in patients undergoing ASCT [23]. Based on the MRD, they divided the homogeneous group of patients in conventional CR into two new groups: one with a high level of MRD and an associated high probability of relapse and a second with low or undetectable MRD and excellent prognosis. This data has been further corroborated in two pivotal studies by the Spanish and UK groups in the context of large multicenter clinical trials. In an analysis of 295 newly diagnosed patients, the Spanish group demonstrated that patients who became MRD negative by MFC at day 100 post-ASCT had a significantly favorable outcome ($P = 0.002$) with progression-free survival (PFS) of 71 months and OS not reached [24]. In contrast, patients who continued to show detectable MRD had a PFS of 37 months and OS of 89 months. Patients with both persistent MRD and high-risk disease had the worst outcome (3-year time to progression: 0% and 3-year OS 32%) [25]. In a very similar analysis evaluating 397 patients from the UK Myeloma IX study with MFC, the MRD was associated with a significantly inferior PFS (15.5 vs. 28.6 months, $P < 0.001$) and OS (59 vs. 80.6 months, $P = 0.018$) [26]. In the intensive pathway, the patient cohorts with different prognoses and was stratified based on combined MRD status and cytogenetic risk group. Median PFS for favorable cytogenetics was 44.2 and 33.7 months for MRD negative and MRD positive, respectively, whereas median PFS for adverse cytogenetics was 15.7 and 8.7 months for MRD negative and MRD positive, respectively [26]. More recently, these observations were reproduced using ASO-PCR [27] and NGS [28], which again corroborated the prognostic value of MRD assessment in transplant-eligible MM patients.

It can be concluded that MRD positivity usually portends adverse prognosis. However, patients achieving MRD negativity also eventually relapse, and at this point we still do not know if we should alter our management for patients per MRD status. Global efforts are underway to standardize and harmonize criteria of automated MRD testing in MM to ensure uniform assessment of response and clinical prognostication. MRD-driven prospective clinical trials (incorporating MRD negativity as primary endpoint) are ongoing to compare and evaluate the efficacy of different treatment strategies, particularly in the consolidation and maintenance settings, and to adapt/modify treatment according to the MRD status. These trials will hopefully provide the rationale for the use of MRD assessment in the future risk stratification schema.

2.6   What About Imaging-Based Response for Risk Stratification?

Sensitive imaging during and after treatment has the potential to improve the definition of MRD and risk stratification by providing information on patchy bone marrow disease and extramedullary sites, complementing MRD assessment in bone marrow sample obtained from single site. MRD-negative patients, who continue to be immunofixation positive or negative, may still have focal lesions or extramedullary sites of active disease. In this respect, lesions that are equivocally positive on MRI or fluorodeoxyglucose-positron emission tomography (FDG-PET) can be subjected to sampling. The application of FDG-PET as a monitoring tool showed that persistence of FDG activity after induction or ASCT was associated with poor PFS and OS. Importantly, 23% of patients who achieved CR but were still positive on PET-CT had significantly shorter 4-year estimate of PFS in comparison with that of PET-negative patients (30% vs. 61%; $P = 0.02$) [29]. In the total therapy (TT) 3 trial for newly diagnosed MM, the presence of more than three FDG-avid focal lesions in the GEP-defined low-risk group served as an independent predictor associated with inferior OS and EFS. The entire high-risk group fared poorly [30]. In addition, this trial showed that a decrease in FDG SUV (max) before ASCT conferred a survival benefit, reflecting the importance of complete suppression of tumor metabolism in MM. Persistence of greater than three focal lesions at day 7 after the start of induction therapy, irrespective of GEP-defined risk, was associated with high risk of relapse or death in TT3A and TT3B clinical trials [31]. Walker and colleagues [32] reported the results of a prospective evaluation of MRI before and after treatment with TT2 trial. They showed that seven or more lesions on MRI in the presence of CA were associated with 5-year OS of 37% as opposed to 76% OS in the absence of both features. Furthermore, resolution of lesions, determined by MRI after therapy predicted for superior OS. Similarly, the Heidelberg group showed that the number of focal lesions on whole body MRI after ASCT is associated with both PFS and OS [33]. Altogether, this indicates that persistence of PET and MRI lesions identifies a group of patients with an inferior response to therapy and that residual focal lesions after treatment may represent the source of relapse. However, it is important to emphasize that focal lesions may show altered signals for several months after therapy, in both responding and nonresponding patients because of treatment-induced necrosis and/or inflammation. Standardization of response definitions by sensitive imaging tools and comparison with bone marrow-based MRD methods, including targeted biopsies, is needed before additional refinements in response criteria based on imaging can be made.

2.7 Do Novel Therapeutics Ameliorate Adverse Impact of High-Risk Cytogenetics?

Over the past 20 years, treatment options for MM have expanded multifold, and the therapies available to patients are more effective. Specifically, IMiDs and proteasome inhibitors (PIs) have contributed to improved PFS and OS and are now considered integral part of treatment before and after ASCT for newly diagnosed patients. Risk stratification has been reviewed in the context of emerging novel therapeutics, distinguishing between therapies that only *improve* the outcomes of high-risk patients when compared with previous therapies vs. those that *overcome* high-risk status, thereby reclassifying these patients as standard risk.

2.7.1 Impact of Proteasome Inhibitors

Most evidence of modifying adverse impact of high-risk cytogenetics in newly diagnosed transplant-eligible patients is available with bortezomib. The data using other approved PIs, i.e., carfilzomib and ixazomib, is not yet mature in frontline setting. Patients with deletion 13 by conventional cytogenetics once considered having high-risk disease, now with the use of bortezomib-based therapies, have an outcome approaching that of intermediate- or standard-risk MM. In a matched-pair analyses of two large phase 2 and 3 trials in relapsed and refractory setting, SUMMIT (Study of Uncontrolled Myeloma Managed With Proteasome Inhibition Therapy) [34] and APEX (Assessment of Proteasome Inhibition for Extending Remissions) [35], Jagannath and colleagues showed that the response and survival were comparable in bortezomib-treated patients with or without del(13) by cytogenetics as an independent prognostic factor [36]. In addition, studies show that historically poor prognostic value associated with del(13/13q) actually stems from its surrogate association with other high-risk features, especially t(4;14) and del(17p) that are concomitantly present in up to 80% of patients harboring del(13/13q) [37].

Whether the novel drugs modify prognostic impact of t(4;14) and del(17p) is still a matter of debate. Chromosomal aberrations t(4:14) and del(17p) have been associated with worse PFS and OS in multivariable analyses independent of ISS stage, even in those undergoing ASCT. These two cytogenetic abnormalities are categorized as high risk based on R-ISS staging. Some, but not all, studies have shown that the negative prognostic implications of t(4;14) and del(17p) can be at least improved (but not overcome) with bortezomib in newly diagnosed transplant-eligible patients.

Notably, this evidence comes from post hoc subgroup analyses of trials that were not specifically targeted or powered for high-risk cytogenetics group.

In HOVON-65/ GMMG-HD4 trial of ASCT, bortezomib as a part of induction and maintenance was compared with VAD (vincristine, doxorubicin, and dexamethasone) induction and thalidomide maintenance [38, 39]. Overall, patients with t(4;14) showed a significantly worse median PFS (21.7 vs. 35.7 months; $P = 0.0002$) and 3-year OS (55% vs. 82%; $P = 0.0003$) compared with patients lacking this aberration. Although the bortezomib arm achieved better results in patients with t(4;14), this did not reach statistical significance. In the same trial, a subgroup analysis of 37 patients with del(17p) demonstrated significantly longer median PFS (26.2 vs. 12.0 months; $P = 0.024$) and improved 3-year OS (69% vs. 17%; $p = 0.028$) in the bortezomib arm than those assigned to VAD. Nonetheless, the 3-year OS of 85% in patients without del(17p) indicates that bortezomib does not completely overcome the adverse prognosis of this abnormality. The IFM group studied the outcome of 507 patients treated with bortezomib and dexamethasone induction before ASCT compared with a cohort of 512 patients treated with VAD [40]. Bortezomib improved both EFS and OS for patients with t(4;14) but not for those with del(17p) when compared with patients treated with VAD induction within the same period.

Two randomized clinical trials evaluated the induction regimen of bortezomib, thalidomide, and dexamethasone (VTD) against thalidomide and dexamethasone (TD) within the context of ASCT and maintenance therapy in newly diagnosed MM. In the trial by Cavo and colleagues, incorporation of VTD before and after double ASCT allowed the adverse effects of t(4;14) to be overcome with improvement in 3-year PFS to 69%. This was analogous to the 3-year PFS of 74% for patients without t(4;14) ($p = 0.66$) [41]. In contrast, patients in the TD arm retained the adverse impact of t(4;14) and experienced comparatively poor 3-year PFS than those without (37% vs. 63%; $p = 0.013$). Benefit was also observed in patients with del(17p13) treated with VTD compared to TD. The median PFS was 12 months in the TD group vs. 22 months in the VTD group ($P = 0.01$). The median OS was 24 months in the TD group vs. not reached at 54 months in the VTD group ($P = 0.003$). In the second trial (Spanish PETHEMA GEM05) where patients received a single course of ASCT and were randomized to thalidomide or interferon alfa-2b or VT maintenance, the cytogenetically defined high-risk group patients including t(4;14) and del(17p13) had a significantly shorter PFS than those with standard risk, irrespective of the treatment [42]. Although high-risk patients had improved median PFS with VTD compared to patients treated with TD (23.5 months vs. 8.9 months, $P = 0.04$), the VTD regimen was not able to overcome the poor prognostic impact of high-risk cytogenetics. This result was in contrast with the Italian study mentioned above. The University of Arkansas TT2 regimen did not include bortezomib and patients with t(4;14) and del(17p) had significantly shorter EFS and OS compared to those without the translocation [43]. This difference disappeared in the bortezomib-containing TT3 regimen, in which bortezomib was added to the induction, consolidation, and maintenance phases of multidrug treatments [44].

In conclusion, it seems that although bortezomib-based regimens improve, to some extent, the PFS and OS in patients with high-risk cytogenetics, this improvement is quite modest and not sufficient to fully overcome the prognosis. A comparison of studies showing favorable results with studies showing less favorable results suggests that the prolonged treatment including bortezomib-based induction therapy before tandem ASCT and bortezomib maintenance may overcome the risk of t(4;14) [45]. Therefore, randomized, prospective clinical trials are needed to resolve whether prolonged bortezomib treatment can truly improve and/or overcome the high-risk impact of del(17p) and t(4;14).

2.7.2   Impact of Immunomodulatory Agents

Thalidomide does not abrogate the adverse effect of t(4;14), t(14;16), t(14;20), and del(17) or del(17p) and gain(1q) in transplant-eligible patients [46]. The benefit of lenalidomide in patients with high-risk cytogenetics undergoing ASCT is less clear. Two recent phase III randomized studies comparing ASCT with standard chemotherapy deserve mention [47, 48]. Newly diagnosed patients aged 65 years or younger in each of these studies were treated with four cycles of Rd induction and subsequent autologous stem cell collection using cyclophosphamide and granulocyte colony-stimulating factor (GCSF) mobilization. Consolidation and maintenance were different in the two studies. Palumbo and colleagues [47] randomized patients to receive consolidation with six cycles of melphalan, prednisone, and lenalidomide (MPR) or two courses of ASCT and maintenance with lenalidomide or no maintenance. Gay and colleagues [48] randomized patients to receive consolidation with six cycles of chemotherapy (cyclophosphamide and Rd) or two courses of ASCT and maintenance with lenalidomide or lenalidomide and prednisone. Both studies showed significantly shorter PFS and OS for the chemotherapy arm compared with the ASCT arm. In a post hoc analysis of patients assigned to chemotherapy, those with high-risk cytogenetic abnormalities had worse PFS (15.7 months vs. 47.1 months) and OS (52% vs. 87%) than did those with standard-risk cytogenetic abnormalities [48]. High-risk was defined by the presence of del(17p), t(4;14), or t(14;16). The difference in PFS between high-risk and standard-risk patients (33.4 months vs. 46.8 months) was less evident with ASCT. In RV-MM-209 trial, patients had insignificant improvement in PFS favoring ASCT for high-risk (HR 0.3, 95% CI 0.37–1.42, $P = 0.40$) and standard-risk group (HR 0.49, 95% CI 0.24–0.62) [47]. Unfortunately, the low number of patients in each subgroup combined with the number of patients not evaluable for cytogenetic risk limited the value of these analyses.

In a study of newly diagnosed MM patients treated with Rd induction, the high-risk group, defined by the presence of hypodiploidy, del(13q), del(17p), t(4;14), t(14;16), or plasma-cell labeling index of 3% or greater, had a shorter PFS (18.5 months vs. 36.5 months $P < 0.001$) and less durable responses compared with standard-risk group. Although the 3-year OS of 77% for high-risk group of patients was not statistically different from OS of 86% for standard risk, $P = 0.4$ [49]. In contrast, in the phase 3 E4A03 study comparing lenalidomide with either high or low-dose dexamethasone in patients with newly diagnosed MM, the 2-year OS in patients with high-risk cytogenetic abnormalities was significantly shorter compared with standard risk (76% vs. 91%, respectively, ($P = 0.004$)) [50]. In both these studies it is not clear how many patients went on to receive ASCT. In the maintenance setting, the Intergroupe Francophone du Myélome (IFM) found that lenalidomide maintenance was associated with an improvement in PFS from 24 to 42 months ($P < 0.0001$). In patients with del(17p), lenalidomide maintenance was associated with an improvement in PFS from 14 to 29 months ($P < 0.02$), but it did not overcome this risk. In patients with t(4;14), the improvement in PFS was from 24 to 28 months ($P < 0.04$) [51].

Therefore, from the available evidence, it can be concluded that there is no clear and consistent evidence of an improvement in PFS or OS with lenalidomide-based induction (Rd or CRd without bortezomib) in high-risk newly diagnosed MM patients undergoing ASCT.

2.8 How Do We Prioritize Treatment for Transplant-Eligible Newly Diagnosed MM According to the Risk Category?

As we move into 2016, early ASCT for all eligible patients remains the standard of care irrespective of risk stratification. In the absence of comparative phase III studies, focused on a risk category, it is challenging to make categorical recommendations regarding the risk-aligned management strategies for transplant-eligible newly diagnosed MM. Besides risk stratification, other factors must always be taken into consideration when prognosticating patients for treatment selection, such as host-related factors (age, performance status, organ function, comprehensive geriatric assessment, and comorbidities) and tumor-related factors (plasma cell proliferation rate, extramedullary disease [EMD], and plasma cell leukemia [PCL]).

Two phase III randomized studies (discussed above) using Rd-based regimens show that PFS is better with early ASCT, but the transplant itself does not provide a meaningful benefit in OS [47, 48]. Missing in these studies was the use of a PI, which is believed to be key to improved survival for high-risk patients. Ongoing large collaborative studies (the European Myeloma Network 02 trial and the IFM/Dana–Farber Cancer Institute 2009 trial; ClinicalTrials.gov numbers NCT01208766, NCT01191060, and NCT01208662) are evaluating effective drug combinations that include a PI and an IMiD vs. ASCT, the benefit of early vs. late transplantation, and the effects of varying the duration of maintenance therapy. At the 2015 American Society of Hematology (ASH) meeting in Orlando, the results from the IFM part of the study were presented, showing that the PFS was longer in the arm with three cycles of RVd followed by upfront ASCT, followed by two additional cycles of RVd and 1 year of lenalidomide maintenance [52]. In the upfront ASCT arm, 93% of patients underwent ASCT, and five toxic deaths occurred during mobilization or in the actual transplant phase (1.4%). ASCT was found to improve PFS (HR 1.5, 95% CI1.2–1.9). The 3-year post-randomization PFS was 61% in the upfront ASCT arm vs. 48% in the delayed ASCT arm. OS was not statistically different between the two arms. In the absence of data confirming the detrimental effect of delayed ASCT, reserving ASCT for future use at disease progression is another treatment option that must be discussed clearly with the patients. The major deterrent to delayed ASCT is the concern that considerable proportion of patients may not continue to be eligible or fit to receive transplantation at the time of relapse, as shown in a study where only 43% of patients (treated with conventional chemotherapy frontline) could receive ASCT at the time of relapse [48].

In the absence of randomized data comparing efficacy, choosing the best induction regimen among a wide range of combinations can be challenging. Depth of response prior to ASCT appears to correlate with the PFS and OS [53]. Three-drug induction incorporating an IMiD and a PI has shown to generate deeper responses than two-drug regimens such as VD or Rd. [54]. The idea is to accelerate and maintain responses given the high risk of genetic instability and propensity to rapidly progress in the face of suboptimal therapy. In real-life practice RVD and VCD (aka CyBorD) are the commonly used regimens in the USA and VTD in other parts of the world. A phase 2 EVOLUTION study suggests that RVD and VCD yield similar results [55]. In a head-to-head comparison within a phase III randomized trial, the overall response rate was significantly higher in the VTD arm, 92.3% vs. 83.4% in the VCD arm ($p = 0.01$), when used as induction prior to ASCT. Similarly, in a retrospective matched pair analysis of patients randomly assigned to the VTD arm of the GIMEMA-MMY-3006 study and patients who received VCD induction in the EMN-02 showed that VTD increased the CR rate three times more than VCD (19 vs. 6%, $P < 0.001$) [56]. This improvement was retained across high-risk cytogenetics as defined by the presence of t(4;14) and/or del(17p) (23% vs. 8%, $P = 0.03$) and among patients with ISS stage II + III (20% vs. 4%, $P < 0.001$). An IMiD and a PI, in combination with dexamethasone, should be the preferred combination, especially for high-risk patients. Because of stringent requirements, older patients and those with comorbidities have generally been excluded from frontline clinical trials. Therefore, information is lacking about how best to manage patients with hepatic or renal failure, preexisting cardiac or vascular disorders, or gastrointestinal and malabsorption syndromes. VCD has been a reasonably safe option for those with suboptimal renal function, with the option to switch to RVD (for high-risk patients) after renal activity is restored. In patients presenting with PCL or extensive EMD, in whom a fast response is required, or for those with rapid progression to induction, more intensive regimens, such as continuous-infusion cisplatin, doxorubicin, cyclophosphamide, and etoposide (PACE), combined with bortezomib or carfilzomib and dexamethasone are used taking adequate prevention measures for tumor lysis syndrome to avoid the risk of irreversible disease complications [57].

Induction treatment is generally continued up to best optimal response, usually 4–6 cycles, after which all transplant-eligible patients proceed with autologous peripheral blood stem cell (PBSC) collection. Stem cells are collected after GCSF and plerixafor mobilization for at least one and usually more than one ASCT. Collecting PBSC early during treatment ensures that stem cells are healthy and are less exposed (both in quantity and quality) to potentially mutagenic therapies.

Newer agents including next-generation PI (carfilzomib, ixazomib), IMiD (pomalidomide), or monoclonal antibodies/immunotherapies (elotuzumab, daratumumab, PD-1/PDL-1 inhibitors) seem to be effective for high-risk MM group in small nonrandomized studies; however systematic studies are being conducted in frontline setting (during induction and/or consolidation) for transplant-eligible patients with high-risk or standard-risk MM, and their results will be important for optimizing regimens.

Tandem ASCT has been shown to improve response for patients achieving less than very good partial response (VGPR) after one ASCT, but these studies were conducted before the use of PI and IMiD. Although tandem ASCT combined with bortezomib-based induction and maintenance may improve PFS in patients with t(4;14) and/or del(17p), this strategy is not routinely implemented as the evidence is not corroborated from stratified randomized studies. Randomized studies comparing early vs. delayed transplant (NCT01208662) or single vs. tandem ASCT (NCT01208766) are ongoing to clarify which populations should proceed for early or tandem ASCT and which population should wait for delayed ASCT.

Lenalidomide (single agent) maintenance until progression is recommended for patients who can tolerate it, based on randomized phase III data and subset analyses proving efficacy in improving PFS for standard-risk patients. For high-risk patients with PCL, t(14;16), del 17(p), and 1q+ or GEP70 score, combined PI and IMID maintenance should be considered because they do not do well with single agent maintenance. In the recent report, VRD maintenance for up to 3 years, followed by single agent lenalidomide maintenance until progression has shown promising results in terms of PFS (median 32 months) and OS (>90% at 3 years) in patients with high-risk cytogenetics [58]. Ongoing studies are examining RVD, carfilzomib-lenalidomide-dexamethasone (KRD), daratumumab, and other new agents in terms of content (single agent vs. combined) and duration (short vs. long) of maintenance therapy.

Allogeneic SCT is not clearly established as a standard treatment approach for most MM patients. In a recent meta-analysis evaluating six trials comparing tandem ASCT vs. ASCT followed by reduced intensity allogeneic SCT, the latter approach was shown to be associated with a higher CR rate and transplant-related mortality without clear benefit in PFS and OS, and the majority of patients relapsed after tandem autologous-allogeneic SCT [59]. For high-risk GEP-70, del(17p), t(4;14), +1q, or plasma cell leukemia, especially with multiple high-risk abnormalities, or in combination with higher stage or high LDH, eligible young patients should be considered for clinical trials examining allogeneic SCT. Novel strategies in the context of allogeneic SCT are being studied that would reduce transplant-related mortality and improve long-term outcomes.

2.9 Summary and Conclusions

Risk stratification at diagnosis is recommended for all patients as it helps with predicting response and in some cases with selecting treatment. Consensus guidelines from the IMWG support a comprehensive cytogenetic and FISH evaluation in all patients with MM at the time of diagnosis and at relapse. FISH panel is used for detection of t(11;14), t(6;14), t(4;14), t(14;16), t(14;20), del(17p13), 1q+, trisomies of odd-numbered chromosomes, and del(1p32). Conventional cytogenetics (karyotyping) is helpful for detection of deletion 13, monosomy 13, or hypodiploidy. Combined models, such as R-ISS, provide improved outcome prognostication and should be routinely adapted in clinic. Risk stratification should continue over time because risk factors can change, thus altering an individual's risk for progression. Studies of GEP are uncovering biological heterogeneity with prognostic significance, and wherever possible GEP data should be collected within or outside of the clinical trials to provide a framework within which newer technologies such as mutational analysis and NGS can be integrated. The use of FDG-PET-CT provides additional predictive information when used at diagnosis and after treatment. There is unequivocal evidence, irrespective of study design, chemotherapy protocol, and MRD measurement method, that MRD is a strong and independent prognostic factor. Future prognostic models in MM are likely to integrate GEP, functional imaging, and MRD within existing risk classification, which would influence the choice of treatment.

Treatment selection based on risk stratification, especially for high-risk patients who constitute about 15–20% of newly diagnosed transplant-eligible population, is an ongoing theme of most clinical trials. Managing high-risk patients continues to be a challenge, and a coordinated effort to put these patients on clinical trials will be required to efficiently determine the optimal therapies. In high-risk MM, highly synergistic combination therapies including next-generation IMiDs and PIs, monoclonal antibodies, and immunotherapy-based approaches are being investigated within the context of induction, consolidation and maintenance regimens, tandem transplantation, second transplantation at the time of relapse, and nonmyeloablative allogeneic stem cell transplantation. Some examples of ongoing studies testing novel strategies in high-risk MM patients include in vivo purging with daratumumab after induction (prior to ASCT), activated marrow infiltrating lymphocytes with ASCT followed by lenalidomide and tadalafil, nonmyeloablative allogeneic transplant followed by bortezomib, matched-donor stem cell transplant using Flu-Bu4, allogeneic transplant using bortezomib given together with Flu-Mel conditioning with or without total marrow irradiation, maintenance ixazomib after allogeneic SCT, and vaccine therapy after ASCT.

In conclusion, there have been significant improvements in the outcomes for patients with MM over the past 20 years related to the use of high-dose melphalan and availability of IMiDs and PIs. The outcome is expected to further improve with emerging therapeutics that target the molecular heterogeneity of the disease. Thus, refining molecular classification and risk classification in MM remains an important goal of ongoing research, so that biology-based individualized treatment can be delivered to many MM patients in the future.

References

1. Chng WJ, Dispenzieri A, Chim CS, Fonseca R, Goldschmidt H, Lentzsch S, et al. IMWG consensus on risk stratification in multiple myeloma. Leukemia. 2014;28(2):269–77.
2. Zhu YX, Braggio E, Shi CX, Bruins LA, Schmidt JE, Van Wier S, et al. Cereblon expression is required for the antimyeloma activity of lenalidomide and pomalidomide. Blood. 2011;118(18):4771–9.
3. Carbone PP, Kellerhouse LE, Gehan EA. Plasmacytic myeloma. A study of the relationship of survival to various clinical manifestations and anomalous protein type in 112 patients. Am J Med. 1967;42(6):937–48.
4. Dawson AA, Ogston D. Factors influencing the prognosis in myelomatosis. Postgrad Med J. 1971;47(552):635–8.
5. Durie BG, Salmon SE. A clinical staging system for multiple myeloma. Correlation of measured myeloma cell mass with presenting clinical features, response to treatment, and survival. Cancer. 1975;36(3):842–54.
6. Cassuto JP, Krebs BP, Viot G, Dujardin P, Masseyeff R. Beta 2 microglobulin, a tumour marker of lymphoproliferative disorder. Lancet. 1978;2(8096):950.
7. Bataille R, Durie BG, Grenier J. Serum beta2 microglobulin and survival duration in multiple myeloma: a simple reliable marker for staging. Br J Haematol. 1983;55(3):439–47.
8. Dewald GW, Kyle RA, Hicks GA, Greipp PR. The clinical significance of cytogenetic studies in 100 patients with multiple myeloma, plasma cell leukemia, or amyloidosis. Blood. 1985;66(2):380–90.
9. Tricot G, Sawyer JR, Jagannath S, Desikan KR, Siegel D, Naucke S, et al. Unique role of cytogenetics in the prognosis of patients with myeloma receiving high-dose therapy and autotransplants. J Clin Oncol. 1997;15(7):2659–66.
10. Fonseca R, Bergsagel PL, Drach J, Shaughnessy J, Gutierrez N, Stewart AK, et al. International Myeloma Working Group molecular classification of multiple myeloma: spotlight review. Leukemia. 2009;23(12):2210–21.
11. Greipp PR, San Miguel J, Durie BG, Crowley JJ, Barlogie B, Blade J, et al. International staging system for multiple myeloma. J Clin Oncol. 2005;23(15):3412–20.
12. Dimopoulos MA, Barlogie B, Smith TL, Alexanian R. High serum lactate dehydrogenase level as a marker for drug resistance and short survival in multiple myeloma. Ann Intern Med. 1991;115(12):931–5.
13. Terpos E, Katodritou E, Roussou M, Pouli A, Michalis E, Delimpasi S, et al. High serum lactate dehydrogenase adds prognostic value to the international myeloma staging system even in the era of novel agents. Eur J Haematol. 2010;85(2):114–9.
14. Zhan F, Hardin J, Kordsmeier B, Bumm K, Zheng M, Tian E, et al. Global gene expression profiling of multiple myeloma, monoclonal gammopathy of undetermined significance, and normal bone marrow plasma cells. Blood. 2002;99(5):1745–57.
15. Shaughnessy JD Jr, Zhan F, Burington BE, Huang Y, Colla S, Hanamura I, et al. A validated gene expression model of high-risk multiple myeloma is defined by deregulated expression of genes mapping to chromosome 1. Blood. 2007;109(6):2276–84.
16. Kuiper R, Broyl A, de Knegt Y, van Vliet MH, van Beers EH, van der Holt B, et al. A gene expression signature for high-risk multiple myeloma. Leukemia. 2012;26(11):2406–13.
17. Decaux O, Lode L, Magrangeas F, Charbonnel C, Gouraud W, Jezequel P, et al. Prediction of survival in multiple myeloma based on gene expression profiles reveals cell cycle and chromosomal instability signatures in high-risk patients and hyperdiploid signatures in low-risk patients: a study of the Intergroupe Francophone du Myelome. J Clin Oncol. 2008;26(29):4798–805.
18. Dickens NJ, Walker BA, Leone PE, Johnson DC, Brito JL, Zeisig A, et al. Homozygous deletion mapping in myeloma samples identifies genes and an expression signature relevant to pathogenesis and outcome. Clin Cancer Res. 2010;16(6):1856–64.
19. Chng WJ, Chung TH, Kumar S, Usmani S, Munshi N, Avet-Loiseau H, et al. Gene signature combinations improve prognostic stratification of multiple myeloma patients. Leukemia. 2015;30(5):1071–8.

20. Palumbo A, Avet-Loiseau H, Oliva S, Lokhorst HM, Goldschmidt H, Rosinol L, et al. Revised international staging system for multiple myeloma: a report from International Myeloma Working Group. J Clin Oncol. 2015;33(26):2863–9.
21. Moreau P, Cavo M, Sonneveld P, Rosinol L, Attal M, Pezzi A, et al. Combination of international scoring system 3, high lactate dehydrogenase, and t(4;14) and/or del(17p) identifies patients with multiple myeloma (MM) treated with front-line autologous stem-cell transplantation at high risk of early MM progression-related death. J Clin Oncol. 2014;32(20):2173–80.
22. Rajkumar SV, Harousseau JL, Durie B, Anderson KC, Dimopoulos M, Kyle R, et al. Consensus recommendations for the uniform reporting of clinical trials: report of the International Myeloma Workshop Consensus Panel 1. Blood. 2011;117(18):4691–5.
23. Rawstron AC, Davies FE, DasGupta R, Ashcroft AJ, Patmore R, Drayson MT, et al. Flow cytometric disease monitoring in multiple myeloma: the relationship between normal and neoplastic plasma cells predicts outcome after transplantation. Blood. 2002;100(9):3095–100.
24. Paiva B, Vidriales MB, Cervero J, Mateo G, Perez JJ, Montalban MA, et al. Multiparameter flow cytometric remission is the most relevant prognostic factor for multiple myeloma patients who undergo autologous stem cell transplantation. Blood. 2008;112(10):4017–23.
25. Paiva B, Gutierrez NC, Rosinol L, Vidriales MB, Montalban MA, Martinez-Lopez J, et al. High-risk cytogenetics and persistent minimal residual disease by multiparameter flow cytometry predict unsustained complete response after autologous stem cell transplantation in multiple myeloma. Blood. 2012;119(3):687–91.
26. Rawstron AC, Child JA, de Tute RM, Davies FE, Gregory WM, Bell SE, et al. Minimal residual disease assessed by multiparameter flow cytometry in multiple myeloma: impact on outcome in the Medical Research Council Myeloma IX Study. J Clin Oncol. 2013;31(20):2540–7.
27. Puig N, Sarasquete ME, Balanzategui A, Martinez J, Paiva B, Garcia H, et al. Critical evaluation of ASO RQ-PCR for minimal residual disease evaluation in multiple myeloma. A comparative analysis with flow cytometry. Leukemia. 2014;28(2):391–7.
28. Martinez-Lopez J, Lahuerta JJ, Pepin F, Gonzalez M, Barrio S, Ayala R, et al. Prognostic value of deep sequencing method for minimal residual disease detection in multiple myeloma. Blood. 2014;123(20):3073–9.
29. Zamagni E, Patriarca F, Nanni C, Zannetti B, Englaro E, Pezzi A, et al. Prognostic relevance of 18-F FDG PET/CT in newly diagnosed multiple myeloma patients treated with up-front autologous transplantation. Blood. 2011;118(23):5989–95.
30. Bartel TB, Haessler J, Brown TL, Shaughnessy JD Jr, van Rhee F, Anaissie E, et al. F18-fluorodeoxyglucose positron emission tomography in the context of other imaging techniques and prognostic factors in multiple myeloma. Blood. 2009;114(10):2068–76.
31. Usmani SZ, Mitchell A, Waheed S, Crowley J, Hoering A, Petty N, et al. Prognostic implications of serial 18-fluoro-deoxyglucose emission tomography in multiple myeloma treated with total therapy 3. Blood. 2013;121(10):1819–23.
32. Walker R, Barlogie B, Haessler J, Tricot G, Anaissie E, Shaughnessy JD Jr, et al. Magnetic resonance imaging in multiple myeloma: diagnostic and clinical implications. J Clin Oncol. 2007;25(9):1121–8.
33. Hillengass J, Ayyaz S, Kilk K, Weber MA, Hielscher T, Shah R, et al. Changes in magnetic resonance imaging before and after autologous stem cell transplantation correlate with response and survival in multiple myeloma. Haematologica. 2012;97(11):1757–60.
34. Richardson PG, Sonneveld P, Schuster MW, Irwin D, Stadtmauer EA, Facon T, et al. Bortezomib or high-dose dexamethasone for relapsed multiple myeloma. N Engl J Med. 2005;352(24):2487–98.
35. Richardson PG, Barlogie B, Berenson J, Singhal S, Jagannath S, Irwin D, et al. A phase 2 study of bortezomib in relapsed, refractory myeloma. N Engl J Med. 2003;348(26):2609–17.
36. Jagannath S, Richardson PG, Sonneveld P, Schuster MW, Irwin D, Stadtmauer EA, et al. Bortezomib appears to overcome the poor prognosis conferred by chromosome 13 deletion in phase 2 and 3 trials. Leukemia. 2007;21(1):151–7.
37. Gutierrez NC, Castellanos MV, Martin ML, Mateos MV, Hernandez JM, Fernandez M, et al. Prognostic and biological implications of genetic abnormalities in multiple myeloma under-

going autologous stem cell transplantation: t(4;14) is the most relevant adverse prognostic factor, whereas RB deletion as a unique abnormality is not associated with adverse prognosis. Leukemia. 2007;21(1):143–50.

38. Sonneveld P, Schmidt-Wolf IG, van der Holt B, El Jarari L, Bertsch U, Salwender H, et al. Bortezomib induction and maintenance treatment in patients with newly diagnosed multiple myeloma: results of the randomized phase III HOVON-65/ GMMG-HD4 trial. J Clin Oncol. 2012;30(24):2946–55.

39. Neben K, Lokhorst HM, Jauch A, Bertsch U, Hielscher T, van der Holt B, et al. Administration of bortezomib before and after autologous stem cell transplantation improves outcome in multiple myeloma patients with deletion 17p. Blood. 2012;119(4):940–8.

40. Avet-Loiseau H, Leleu X, Roussel M, Moreau P, Guerin-Charbonnel C, Caillot D, et al. Bortezomib plus dexamethasone induction improves outcome of patients with t(4;14) myeloma but not outcome of patients with del(17p). J Clin Oncol. 2010;28(30):4630–4.

41. Cavo M, Tacchetti P, Patriarca F, Petrucci MT, Pantani L, Galli M, et al. Bortezomib with thalidomide plus dexamethasone compared with thalidomide plus dexamethasone as induction therapy before, and consolidation therapy after, double autologous stem-cell transplantation in newly diagnosed multiple myeloma: a randomised phase 3 study. Lancet. 2010;376(9758):2075–85.

42. Rosinol L, Oriol A, Teruel AI, Hernandez D, Lopez-Jimenez J, de la Rubia J, et al. Superiority of bortezomib, thalidomide, and dexamethasone (VTD) as induction pretransplantation therapy in multiple myeloma: a randomized phase 3 PETHEMA/GEM study. Blood. 2012;120(8):1589–96.

43. Barlogie B, Anaissie E, van Rhee F, Haessler J, Hollmig K, Pineda-Roman M, et al. Incorporating bortezomib into upfront treatment for multiple myeloma: early results of total therapy 3. Br J Haematol. 2007;138(2):176–85.

44. Pineda-Roman M, Zangari M, Haessler J, Anaissie E, Tricot G, van Rhee F, et al. Sustained complete remissions in multiple myeloma linked to bortezomib in total therapy 3: comparison with total therapy 2. Br J Haematol. 2008;140(6):625–34.

45. Sonneveld P, Goldschmidt H, Rosinol L, Blade J, Lahuerta JJ, Cavo M, et al. Bortezomib-based versus nonbortezomib-based induction treatment before autologous stem-cell transplantation in patients with previously untreated multiple myeloma: a meta-analysis of phase III randomized, controlled trials. J Clin Oncol. 2013;31(26):3279–87.

46. Sonneveld P, Avet-Loiseau H, Lonial S, Usmani S, Siegel D, Anderson KC, et al. Treatment of Multiple Myeloma with high-risk cytogenetics: a consensus of the International Myeloma Working Group. Blood. 2016;127(24):2955–62.

47. Palumbo A, Cavallo F, Gay F, Di Raimondo F, Ben Yehuda D, Petrucci MT, et al. Autologous transplantation and maintenance therapy in multiple myeloma. N Engl J Med. 2014;371(10):895–905.

48. Gay F, Oliva S, Petrucci MT, Conticello C, Catalano L, Corradini P, et al. Chemotherapy plus lenalidomide versus autologous transplantation, followed by lenalidomide plus prednisone versus lenalidomide maintenance, in patients with multiple myeloma: a randomised, multicentre, phase 3 trial. Lancet Oncol. 2015;16(16):1617–29.

49. Kapoor P, Kumar S, Fonseca R, Lacy MQ, Witzig TE, Hayman SR, et al. Impact of risk stratification on outcome among patients with multiple myeloma receiving initial therapy with lenalidomide and dexamethasone. Blood. 2009;114(3):518–21.

50. Jacobus SJ, Kumar S, Uno H, Van Wier SA, Ahmann GJ, Henderson KJ, et al. Impact of high-risk classification by FISH: an eastern cooperative oncology group (ECOG) study E4A03. Br J Haematol. 2011;155(3):340–8.

51. Attal M, Lauwers-Cances V, Marit G, Caillot D, Moreau P, Facon T, et al. Lenalidomide maintenance after stem-cell transplantation for multiple myeloma. N Engl J Med. 2012;366(19):1782–91.

52. Attal M, Lauwers-Cances V, Hulin C, Facon T, Caillot D, Escoffre M, et al. Autologous transplantation for multiple myeloma in the era of new drugs: a phase III study of the Intergroupe Francophone Du Myelome (IFM/DFCI 2009 Trial). Blood. 2015;126(23):391.

53. Martinez-Lopez J, Blade J, Mateos MV, Grande C, Alegre A, Garcia-Larana J, et al. Long-term prognostic significance of response in multiple myeloma after stem cell transplantation. Blood. 2011;118(3):529–34.
54. Moreau P, Attal M, Facon T. Frontline therapy of multiple myeloma. Blood. 2015;125(20):3076–84.
55. Kumar S, Flinn I, Richardson PG, Hari P, Callander N, Noga SJ, et al. Randomized, multicenter, phase 2 study (EVOLUTION) of combinations of bortezomib, dexamethasone, cyclophosphamide, and lenalidomide in previously untreated multiple myeloma. Blood. 2012;119(19):4375–82.
56. Cavo M, Pantani L, Pezzi A, Petrucci MT, Patriarca F, Di Raimondo F, et al. Bortezomib-thalidomide-dexamethasone (VTD) is superior to bortezomib-cyclophosphamide-dexamethasone (VCD) as induction therapy prior to autologous stem cell transplantation in multiple myeloma. Leukemia. 2015;29(12):2429–31.
57. Usmani SZ, Rodriguez-Otero P, Bhutani M, Mateos MV, Miguel JS. Defining and treating high-risk multiple myeloma. Leukemia. 2015;29(11):2119–25.
58. Nooka AK, Kaufman JL, Muppidi S, Langston A, Heffner LT, Gleason C, et al. Consolidation and maintenance therapy with lenalidomide, bortezomib and dexamethasone (RVD) in high-risk myeloma patients. Leukemia. 2014;28(3):690–3.
59. Armeson KE, Hill EG, Costa LJ. Tandem autologous vs autologous plus reduced intensity allogeneic transplantation in the upfront management of multiple myeloma: meta-analysis of trials with biological assignment. Bone Marrow Transplant. 2013;48(4):562–7.
60. Neben K, Jauch A, Bertsch U, Heiss C, Hielscher T, Seckinger A, et al. Combining information regarding chromosomal aberrations t(4;14) and del(17p13) with the International Staging System classification allows stratification of myeloma patients undergoing autologous stem cell transplantation. Haematologica. 2010;95(7):1150–7.
61. Boyd KD, Ross FM, Chiecchio L, Dagrada GP, Konn ZJ, Tapper WJ, et al. A novel prognostic model in myeloma based on co-segregating adverse FISH lesions and the ISS: analysis of patients treated in the MRC Myeloma IX trial. Leukemia. 2012;26(2):349–55.
62. Avet-Loiseau H, Durie BG, Cavo M, Attal M, Gutierrez N, Haessler J, et al. Combining fluorescent in situ hybridization data with ISS staging improves risk assessment in myeloma: an International Myeloma Working Group collaborative project. Leukemia. 2013;27(3):711–7.
63. Fonseca R, Van Wier SA, Chng WJ, Ketterling R, Lacy MQ, Dispenzieri A, et al. Prognostic value of chromosome 1q21 gain by fluorescent in situ hybridization and increase CKS1B expression in myeloma. Leukemia. 2006;20(11):2034–40.
64. Avet-Loiseau H, Attal M, Campion L, Caillot D, Hulin C, Marit G, et al. Long-term analysis of the IFM 99 trials for myeloma: cytogenetic abnormalities [t(4;14), del(17p), 1q gains] play a major role in defining long-term survival. J Clin Oncol. 2012;30(16):1949–52.

Risk Stratification in Newly Diagnosed Transplant Ineligible Multiple Myeloma

Massimo Offidani, Laura Corvatta, Silvia Gentili,
Elena Aghemo, Antonio Palumbo, Laura Maracci,
and Alessandra Larocca

3.1   Introduction

Multiple myeloma (MM) is a plasma cell disease of older adults, with a median age at diagnosis of ≥ 70 years. The population is rapidly aging, and this phenomenon will lead to a considerable increase in the incidence of MM in the older population in the near future [1, 2].

The introduction of novel agents in the therapeutic armamentarium in the last 15 years has dramatically improved the outcome of MM [3–5]. Nevertheless, in population-based studies, this improvement seems to be rather limited in patients older than 70 years compared with younger patients [3, 6]. The clinical and biological heterogeneity of the MM, together with aging heterogeneity, represents a major challenge in the treatment of elderly MM patients. The appropriate assessment of aging remains an unsolved issue, and this most likely accounts for the gap between outcomes in younger and in older MM patients. Although the disease characteristics reflecting the biology of MM clone and tumor burden seem to be quite similar in young and elderly MM, host factors are very different in the two age groups and play a central role in the tolerability and discontinuation of therapies. Indeed, the

M. Offidani (✉)
Clinica di Ematologia Azienda Ospedaliero- Universitaria Ospedali Riuniti di Ancona, Via Conca, 71, 60020, Ancona, Italy
e-mail: Massimo.Offidani@ospedaliriuniti.marche.it

L. Corvatta • S. Gentili • L. Maracci
Clinica di Ematologia, AOU Ospedali Riuniti di Ancona, Ancona, Italy

E. Aghemo • A. Larocca • A. Palumbo
Myeloma Unit, Division of Hematology, University of Torino, Azienda Ospedaliero- Universitaria Città della Salute e della Scienza di Torino, Via Genova 3, 10126 Torino, Italy
e-mail: appalumbo@yahoo.com

© Springer International Publishing AG 2018
S.Z. Usmani, A.K. Nooka (eds.), *Personalized Therapy for Multiple Myeloma*,
https://doi.org/10.1007/978-3-319-61872-2_3

rate of adverse events leading to dose reductions or therapy interruption is higher in the elderly population; moreover, a population-based study showed that two thirds of early mortality cases occurred in patients older than 70 years [7].

Quality of life (QoL) preservation should be a major endpoint for all patients with MM, but it is particularly relevant in older patients, in whom prolongation of progression-free survival (PFS) and overall survival (OS) cannot be the priority. Nevertheless, QoL of patients with MM depends on disease symptoms as well as on adverse events due to therapy. In this view, response to therapy and tolerability of all drugs administered (including supportive care) is equally highly relevant. In addition, achieving a complete remission (CR) was demonstrated to be closely associated with longer PFS and OS also in older patients [8].

In younger patients, clinical and biological heterogeneity of MM translated into a variable response to treatment and outcome. In older patients, a wide variety of host factors have a strong influence on treatment outcome. Therefore, besides choosing the most effective therapy based on disease-risk stratification, we need appropriate models to recognize patients who are able to tolerate intensive therapy in order to maximize outcome and patients who require a gentler approach to minimize toxicity.

There is growing evidence supporting the concept that chronologic age cannot represent the complexity associated with aging. Other strategies and tools, such as performance status, the presence of comorbidity, geriatric evaluation, and functional, cognitive, and psychosocial status assessments should be considered. The combination of these factors allows a better selection of appropriate, tailored treatments.

In this chapter, we have summarized the data available to stratify elderly patients with MM according to tumor-related characteristics as well as host factors, with the ultimate aim to better define the current status of personalized therapy in the elderly MM population.

3.2   Therapy Overview in Elderly MM Patients

3.2.1   Randomized Phase III Studies

Several randomized studies and a meta-analysis [9] demonstrated that melphalan, prednisone, and thalidomide (MPT) combination was superior to melphalan-prednisone (MP) in terms of response rate, PFS, and OS. Based on these results, MPT was thus considered as the first new standard of care in elderly MM patients since the 1960s. However, MPT was not well tolerated, particularly because of peripheral neuropathy occurring in almost all patients. A randomized study, the VISTA trial [10] demonstrated that bortezomib-melphalan-prednisone (VMP) was unequivocally superior to MP in response rate as well in PFS and OS. Based on that study, VMP was also considered a new standard of care for patients ineligible for transplantation in Europe. Although no direct comparison between MPT and VMP has been performed, one retrospective study demonstrated that VMP was associated with better response rate, tolerability, PFS, and OS [11]. The major drawback of bortezomib is peripheral neuropathy, which can significantly be reduced through the subcutaneous administration instead of standard intravenous injection [12] and the once weekly instead of the twice-weekly schedule [13]. VMP was subsequently compared with VMPT followed by bortezomib-thalidomide maintenance (VMPT-VT) [14, 15]. Results were significantly in favor of VMPT-VT in terms of PFS and OS. Unfortunately, the advantage with this more intensive regimen was less evident in patients older than 75 years, as they frequently discontinued therapy because of toxicity. The Spanish group compared VMP with VTP both followed by VT or VP as maintenance therapy [16]. The two regimens were equivalent in response and survival but, both in induction and in maintenance, the thalidomide-containing regimens (VTP and VT) were significantly worse tolerated. The same group performed a randomized study comparing alternating six courses VMP and six courses of lenalidomide-dexamethasone (Rd) with six sequential courses of VMP followed by six cycles of Rd [17]. To date, no differences were found between the two treatment strategies. Randomized phase III studies comparing VMP with VMP-Daratumumab (an anti-CD38 monoclonal antibody) are ongoing. The safety of VMP-Daratumumab has been investigated in a phase Ib study [18] in which daratumumab was combined with three backbone MM therapies, namely, VD, VTD, and VMP. VMP plus daratumumab was administered to eight elderly patients with a median age of 72 years (range 67–78) inducing an overall response rate (ORR) of 100% and a very good partial response (VGPR) of 50%. Daratumumab did not add to the toxicity of VMP, and no patient discontinued treatment due to adverse events.

Similarly to thalidomide and bortezomib, lenalidomide was tested in combination with MP (MPR) and compared with MPR followed by lenalidomide maintenance (MPR-R) and MP [19]. Patients treated with MPR-R achieved a significantly longer PFS compared with those treated with MP, but this advantage did not translate into a better survival because patients aged 75 years or more frequently had to reduce or to discontinue therapy for toxicity. However, all patients, including very elderly ones, did benefit from maintenance therapy with lenalidomide. Recently, MPR-R was randomly compared with MPT-T [20]. No differences in PFS and OS between two treatment arms were seen, while MPR-R was more tolerated, particularly in terms of peripheral neuropathy and hematological toxicity. Yet, there were no differences in the rate of patients who completed the six cycles of therapy between regimens, and no differences were detected between age groups of ≤75 and >75 within each regimen. To reduce toxicity, a lower dose of melphalan (5 mg/m^2 instead of 9 mg/m^2) was associated to lenalidomide and prednisone (mPR). This combination was compared to MPT, and no differences were found for the main outcome measures [21]. Despite the advantages, the results reported in the above trials hampered MPR-R to become a new standard therapy.

3.2.2   Phase II Studies

A modified regimen of bortezomib-lenalidomide-dexamethasone compared with the one used in young patients (RVD lite: bortezomib 1.3 mg/m^2 weekly, lenalidomide 15 mg/day on days 1–21, and dexamethasone 20 mg twice weekly if ≤75 years or once weekly if >75 years) was evaluated in a phase II study in elderly patients [22]. Ninety percent of the 30 patients enrolled obtained response, 53% achieved a VGPR, and therapy seemed to be well tolerated also in older patients.

Carfilzomib, the second-in-class proteasome inhibitor, was recently tested in association with melphalan and prednisone (CMP) in a dose-escalating phase I/II study [23] which enrolled 72 patients with a median age of 72 years (range 66–86 years). Patients received a median of nine cycles of CMP, and at least a partial response (PR) was reported in 90% of them, including 58% achieving at least VGPR and 12% a complete response (CR). After a median follow-up of 22 months, the projected 3-year OS was 80%. CMP combination showed a good safety profile, less than 5% of patients developed grade 3–4 non hematologic toxicities and, remarkably, grade 3 peripheral neuropathy occurred only in one of 68 patients. The results of randomized phase III study comparing VMP with CMP are awaited.

Carfilzomib, administered either twice weekly or once weekly, was tested in combination with cyclophosphamide and dexamethasone (CCyD) in phase II studies including elderly patients. In the first study [24], 58 patients received nine 4-week cycles of CCyD (with carfilzomib given on days 1, 2, 8, 9, 15, 16 at 20 mg/m^2 on days 1, 2 of cycle 1 and 36 mg/m^2 thereafter) followed by maintenance with carfilzomib until disease progression or intolerance. The ORR was 95%, including 71% at least a VGPR and 49% near CR (nCR). After a median follow-up of 18 months, the 2-year PFS and OS rates were 76% and 87%, respectively. The most common grade 3–4 toxicities were neutropenia (20%), anemia (11%), and cardiopulmonary events (7%), while no severe peripheral neuropathy was reported. In the second phase II study [25], carfilzomib at dose of 70 mg/m^2 on days 1, 8, and 15 was administered in combination with cyclophosphamide and dexamethasone. Forty-seven patients were enrolled; the median age was 72 years. After a median of six cycles, 80% achieved at least a PR, 60% at least a VGPR, and 28% CR/nCR. Main grade 3–4 side effects were neutropenia (22%), infections (10%), thrombocytopenia (7%), and acute pulmonary edema (5%), and no peripheral neuropathy was reported.

The combination of carfilzomib, lenalidomide, and low-dose dexamethasone (CRd) was explored in a phase I/II study [26] which enrolled 23 patients. They received eight 28-day CRd induction cycles (carfilzomib with escalating doses from 20 to 36 mg/m^2 on days 1, 2, 8, 9, 15, and 16; lenalidomide 25 mg/day on days 1–21 and dexamethasone 40 mg on days 1, 8, 15, 22 for cycles 1–4 and at 20 mg thereafter), followed by sixteen 28-day CRd maintenance cycles (carfilzomib 36 mg/m^2 on days 1, 2, 15, and 16, lenalidomide, and dexamethasone given at the same dosage and schedule). After 24 cycles, a single agent maintenance with lenalidomide was provided off protocol. All patients achieved at least a PR, including 65% of patients with stringent CR (sCR). This association led to 3-year PFS and OS rates of 79.6% and 100%, respectively. The regimen was well tolerated. The main severe toxicities during induction were hematologic, in particular thrombocytopenia (39%) and lymphopenia (35%), while the majority of adverse events reported during maintenance were grades 1–2.

Ixazomib, a new oral proteasome inhibitor, was combined with Rd in a phase II study [27] including a total of 50 patients. Median age was 65 years, but half of patients were ≥65 years old and 18% aged 75 years or over. Most frequent grade 3–4 adverse events were skin disorders (14%), neutropenia (14%), fatigue (12%) and thrombocytopenia (8%). Among 24 evaluable patients aged 65 years or older,

ORR was 88% (38% CR or nCR, 33% VGPR, 17% PR) with a 1-year PFS of 73% and 1-year OS of 83%.

In a phase II study [28], 70 transplant-ineligible MM patients were treated with once-weekly ixazomib 4.0 mg, dexamethasone, and cyclophosphamide 300 or 400 mg/m^2. Preliminary analysis of 30 patients treated at each cyclophosphamide dose showed that 27% of patients treated in the 300 mg/m^2 arm and 23% in the 400 mg/m^2 arm achieved a CR or a VGPR; the ORR was 80% and 73%, respectively. Grade 1–2 peripheral neuropathy was similar in the 300 mg/m^2 and 400 mg/m^2 dose groups (17% and 21%, respectively), with no cases of grade ≥3 peripheral neuropathy. Rates of adverse events were higher with 400 mg/m^2 vs. 300 mg/m^2 cyclophosphamide. Therefore, a lower dose level of cyclophosphamide may be suitable for older patients.

3.2.3 Doublet Vs. Triplet Therapies

Recently, the results of the FIRST in which continuous Rd was compared with MPT and with Rd for 18 months have been published [29, 30]. Continuous Rd was significantly superior to MPT in terms of PFS and OS, including the subgroup of patients older than 75 years (4-year OS: 52% vs. 39%). The rates of therapy reduction or discontinuation were similar in patients aged 65–75 years and those older than that (37% vs. 44% and 21% vs. 26%). Results of two phase III randomized studies comparing Rd with Rd-Elotuzumab and with Rd-Daratumumab are awaited.

Another randomized study [31] compared Rd (lenalidomide 25 mg days 1–21, dexamethasone 40 mg weekly or 20 mg weekly if >75 years) with MPR (melphalan 0.18 mg/kg days 1–4; 0.13 mg/kg if age > 75 years, lenalidomide 10 mg days 1–21, prednisone 1.5 mg/kg days 1–4) and with CPR (cyclophosphamide 50 mg days 1–21, lenalidomide 25 mg days 1–21, prednisone 1.5 mg/kg days 1–4). Six hundred and sixty patients were enrolled, and 38% were older than 75 years. The ORR and VGPR were quite similar, and the three regimens induced comparable median PFS (21, 24, 20 months, respectively) and 4-year OS (58%, 65%, 68%, respectively). No differences were found between patients aged ≤75 and >75 years. However, severe hematological toxicity, infections, and lenalidomide and melphalan reduction and therapy discontinuation were significantly higher in the MPR arm. The IMWG frailty score was retrospectively applied, and 28% of patients were classified as frail. However, there were no differences between fit and frail patients regarding PFS, whereas OS was significantly longer in fit patients.

In the randomized phase IIIb Upfront trial [32], the authors prospectively compared bortezomib-dexamethasone (VD), bortezomib-thalidomide-dexamethasone (VTD), and VMP followed by bortezomib consolidation as frontline therapy in 502 transplant-ineligible patients in a community-based setting. Almost 50% of patients had at least one comorbidity, 42% were ≥75 years old, and 18% aged ≥80 years. VD doublet therapy showed to be as effective as VTD and VMP (CR/nCR: 30%, 40%, 32%, respectively) but less toxic and associated with lower discontinuation rate. With a median follow-up of 42.7 months, the median PFS was 14.7, 15.4, and

17.3 months, respectively. Notably, similar results were observed in terms of OS among the three regimens (global $P = 0.79$).

3.2.4   Adapted Therapies in Older Patients

Few studies addressed the issue of adapted therapy in elderly patients. A phase II trial [33] assessed the combination MPR in 46 unfit elderly myeloma patients (median age 75 years). They received four cycles of lenalidomide and prednisone every 4 weeks, followed by six cycles of MPR consolidation cycles and maintenance with lenalidomide plus prednisone. The PR rate was 80%, including 29% of patients with at least a VGPR. The median PFS and 2-year OS rate was 18.4 months and 80%, respectively. At the maximum tolerated dose during the consolidation (melphalan 25 mg/month and lenalidomide 10 mg/day), the major hematologic toxicity was neutropenia (36.4% grade 3–4), and non-hematologic toxicities included cutaneous reactions (18%) and infections (12%).

In a phase III randomized study [34], VMP was compared with bortezomib-prednisone (VP) and with bortezomib-cyclophosphamide-prednisone (VCP) in an older population of naïve MM. Median age was 77 years, and 66% of patients were frail according to IMWG frailty score. Bortezomib was administered subcutaneously at 1.3 mg/m^2 weekly, whereas melphalan (2 mg), cyclophosphamide (50 mg), and prednisone (25 mg) were given three times a week. All regimens were administered for nine 28-day courses followed by bortezomib every 2 weeks as maintenance therapy. Response rate was similar among the three regimens (86% for VMP vs. 64% vs. 67% for VP and VCP, respectively), including in frail patients. The median PFS and OS were similar among the three groups of patients as well. However, grade 3–5 non-hematologic adverse events, particularly infections and cardiac events, were more frequent in patients receiving VMP. A subgroup analysis by frailty showed that 44% frail patients vs. 39% unfit and 30% fit patients developed at least one grade 3 or higher non-hematologic adverse event, leading to treatment discontinuation in 26% vs. 21% and 11% of patients, respectively. Moreover frail patients had a significantly shorter OS if compared with fit ones (HR 5.57; $p = 0.019$).

3.3   Stratification by Disease-Related Characteristics

Multiple myeloma is a malignancy characterized by large clinical and biological heterogeneity translating into variable responses to treatment and different survival outcomes. Increased therapeutic armamentarium and more effective regimens have led to a better outcome in elderly MM patients, and a further increase in approved therapeutic agents is expected in the coming years. However, considering that a universal approach that is successful in all patients is unlikely to be found due to the high patient heterogeneity, an adequate prognostication to dissect such heterogeneity and to allow a rational choice of treatment is crucial. Several disease-related markers are used today for risk stratification, and they are associated with the biological characteristics of myeloma as cytogenetic and disease burden and with the responsiveness to treatment. Hopefully, biology-based personalized therapy will be available in the future.

3.3.1   Cytogenetic Abnormalities

Most studies on the incidence of chromosomal abnormalities and their prognostic role in MM have been performed in young patients [35, 36] who underwent ASCT, and results are controversial [37]. However, according to IMWG recommendations the term "high risk" should be used in the presence of either del(4;14) or del(17p) detected by FISH, "low risk" in the absence of del(4;14), del(17p), and gain 1q, whereas the term "standard risk" should be adopted for all the remaining patients. Some studies focused on genetic aberrations and their impact on outcome in elderly MM patients. One study [38] found a different distribution of cytogenetic features between patients aged ≤ 61 and ≥ 62 years ($p = 0.02$) with hyperdiploidy being more common in older patients. A retrospective analysis of a large cohort of the French Intergroupe Francophone du Myelome (IFM) [39] including 1890 patients (median age 72 years, range 66–94 years) assessed the incidence and clinical significance of chromosomal abnormalities in two groups of patients, those aged 66 to 75 years and those older than 75 years. The incidence of del(13) and t(4;14) was significantly lower in the older population. This was confirmed when the comparison included not only the cohort of patients aged between 66 and 75 years, but also patients younger than 66 years in whom del(13) incidence was 45% vs. 43.6% vs. 37% in the two older groups ($p = 0.004$), whereas t(4;14) was detected in 14.3%, 10.9%, and 8.3% ($p < 0.001$). In contrast, the incidence of del(17p) was stable within the three groups (6%, 5.9%, and 6.1%, respectively; $p = NS$). Most patients were treated with MPT (40%), and the remaining received MP (22%), VMP (8%), Rd (11%), and high/intermediate-dose melphalan (19%). Independently of the treatment administered, t(4;14) and del(17p) were predictors of shorter PFS and OS. The median PFS for patients who had t(4;14) and del(17p) was 14 ($p < 0.001$) and 11 months ($p < 0.001$), respectively, compared with 24 months for patients who did not have such abnormalities. The respective median OS was 32 ($p < 0.001$) and 19 months ($p < 0.001$) as compared with 50 months. Moreover, the results were similar in elderly and very elderly subgroups. This study demonstrated that in elderly patients, these two chromosomal abnormalities retained the same prognostic value as for younger subjects. In a recent analysis [40] examining a large series of elderly patients with newly diagnosed MM enrolled in a phase III trial comparing VMPT-VT with VMP, the incidence of chromosome 1 aberrations, defined as del(1p) and/or gain(1q), was 50.7%. Multivariate logistic regression analysis performed to evaluate protective/risk factors for the presence of abnormal chromosome 1 identified del(13) ($OR = 1.8$; $p = 0.074$) and t(4;14)/t(14;16) ($OR = 2.06$; $p = 0.051$) to be independent risk factors of borderline significance, while t(11;14) emerged as having a strong protective role ($OR = 0.15$; $p = 0.001$). Moreover, abnormal chromosome 1 was an adverse prognostic factor for both PFS and OS.

The capability of novel agents such as thalidomide, bortezomib, and lenalidomide to overcome the poor prognostic impact of high-risk cytogenetics was retrospectively explored. In the MRC IX trial [41], there was a possible emergence of a late-survival benefit favoring attenuated cyclophosphamide-thalidomide-dexamethasone (CTDa) regimen over MP in patients with unfavorable FISH profile defined as gain(1q), t(4;14), t(14;20), t(14;16), and del(17p). However, in these high-risk patients, thalidomide maintenance was found to have a negative effect on OS (median 35 vs. 47 months; $p = 0.01$). In the Italian phase III trial [42] comparing VMPT-VT with VMP, the outcome of high-risk patients, defined by the presence of t(4;14 t(14;16) or del(17p), was similar in those receiving VMPT-VT or VMP, whereas the outcome of standard-risk patients was superior with VMPT-VT. However, a retrospective analysis of patients enrolled in this trial [40] showed that thalidomide, even if combined with bortezomib, exerts a negative effect on OS in patients with del(17p) as well as in those with abnormal chromosome 1.

In the VISTA trial [43], VMP showed to overcome the adverse prognosis of high-risk cytogenetics since no significant differences were documented between standard- and high-risk patients in terms of 3-year OS, which was 71% in the former and 56% in the latter group (HR 1.346; $p = 0.399$). Nevertheless, due to the small number of patients with unfavorable cytogenetics as t(4;14), t(14;16) and del(17p) ($n = 26$) treated with VMP, no definitive conclusions can be drawn about the impact of bortezomib on high-risk cytogenetic features. Different results were reported in another study by the Spanish group [44] in which patients 65 years of age and older were randomized to receive induction with VMP or VTP and, subsequently, after six cycles, were randomized again to maintenance therapy with VP or VT. Although the response rate after induction was similar in the standard- and high-risk subgroups of patients, after a median follow-up of 32 months, high-risk patients had a significantly shorter PFS compared with standard-risk patients (median 24 months vs. 32 months; HR 1.5; $p = 0.04$) translating into a worse OS (3-year OS: 55% vs. 77%; HR 2.3; $p = 0.001$). Moreover, non-hyperdiploidy patients had a significantly shorter OS compared with hyperdiploidy cases (3-year OS: 63% vs. 77%; $p = 0.04$), and the negative impact of non-hyperdiploidy features resulted more evident in patients receiving VTP as induction suggesting a favorable effect of alkylating included in VMP combination.

Data regarding the impact of cytogenetics with lenalidomide treatment can be drawn from the FIRST trial [29] in which 1623 patients ineligible for autologous stem cell transplantation (ASCT) were randomized to Rd continuously, Rd for 18 cycles, or MPT. In a subgroup analysis presented at the 2015 ASH meeting [45], Rd continuously resulted in a 28% reduced risk of death versus MPT overall and 34% reduced risk in patients without high-risk cytogenetics; the 3-year OS of patients treated with Rd continuously was 40.7% in high risk vs. 77% in not high-risk patients. Similarly, the 3-year PFS was 3% in high-risk patients receiving continuous Rd and MPT compared with 45% and 25.5% in not high-risk patients treated with continuous Rd and MPT, respectively.

Recently, among 240 newly diagnosed patients treated upfront with Rd [46], a cohort of 33 exceptional responders was identified, and they were characterized by a trisomic form of MM. In a retrospective analysis including 484 patients of all ages with newly diagnosed MM by Kumar et al. [47], trisomy of at least one of the odd-numbered chromosome (3, 7, 9, 11, 13, 15, or 17) was observed in 57% of patients. Forty-eight percent of them had trisomy of at least two of the odd-numbered chromosomes which is conventionally termed as hyperdiploidy.

In summary, in elderly MM patients, bortezomib appears to be able to overcome the poor prognosis conferred by t(4;14) and t(14;16) but not that related associated with del(17p) and chromosome 1 aberrations; whereas the benefit of lenalidomide plus dexamethasone seems to be questionable in patients with high-risk cytogenetic features. Second-generation proteasome inhibitors such as carfilzomib and ixazomib, novel immunomodulatory agents such as pomalidomide, and monoclonal antibodies like elotuzumab and daratumumab have been evaluated; preliminary data of carfilzomib combined with cyclophosphamide and dexamethasone (CCyd) in newly diagnosed MM ≥ 65 years of age showed a slightly higher risk of progression in patients with high-risk chromosomal abnormalities (HR 1.85; 95%CI, 0.59–5.85) [24].

3.3.2   Combined International Staging System and FISH/Gene-Expression Profiling Classifiers

The International Staging System (ISS) is based on easy-to-use variables, namely, serum β2-microglobulin and albumin, and represents a major advance in the prognostic stratification. Although in the large international data set used to build this model, patients aged over 65 years had poorer survival than younger patients; ISS demonstrated its applicability also in the older population [48]. However, this staging system has two major limitations: it was developed in the old drugs era, and it does not incorporate cytogenetic or molecular features.

The prognostic assessment can be improved in terms of PFS and OS by combining both t(4;14) and del(17p) detected by FISH analysis along with ISS stage [49]. In the ISS-FISH model, there was a clear impact of age when patients were stratified into younger than 65 years and older than that. OS was longer in patients under the age of 65 years, with ISS stage I or II, no t(4;14) nor del(17p), with a 4-year OS estimate of 75%; whereas outcome was poorer in patients ≥65 years with ISS stage III with either t(4;14) or del(17p), showing a 4-year OS estimate of 24%. However, no patients included in this retrospective study received bortezomib or lenalidomide as frontline treatment.

A new staging system including ISS, chromosomal abnormalities (CA), and serum lactate dehydrogenase (LDH) (R-ISS) has been recently published [50]. This new risk-stratification model has been developed in a large sample size of 3060 patients including both young and elderly patients, and, in contrast with abovementioned studies, all patients were treated with new drugs such as immunomodulatory agents or proteasome inhibitors in association with conventional chemotherapy. Subgroup analyses for PFS and OS confirmed the prognostic role of R-ISS in patients younger and older than 65 years. Patients aged over 65 years with R-ISS III (ISS III, high-risk CA defined as the presence of del(17p) and/or t(4;14) and/or t(14;16) detected by FISH and/or high LDH level) had a median OS of 42 months compared with not reached in patients with R-ISS I (ISS I, no high-risk CA and normal LDH). Moreover, R-ISS retained its prognostic significance regardless of treatment administered upfront.

Recently, different risk groups have been identified by using gene-expression profiling (GEP). The University of Arkansas for Medical Science (UAMS) [51] conducted a study in a population of MM patients including those older than 65 years and found a set of 70 genes able to identify patients at high risk for early disease-related death, representing a 14% of the patient population. A multivariate discriminant analysis found that among the 70 original genes, 17 probe sets could be used to detect high-risk MM patients having a median OS of 3 years. Using GEPs obtained from newly diagnosed patients enrolled in the HOVON65/GMMG-HD4 trial, Kuiper et al. [52] built a prognostic signature of 92 genes (EMC92) whose performance was confirmed in four independent validation data sets including MRC-IX data from both transplant-eligible and -ineligible patients. In the transplant-ineligible setting, patients defined as high risk by the EMC92-gene signature showed a median OS of 18.6 months compared with 33.3 months in standard-risk patients (HR = 2.38). ISS combined with EMC92 [53] allowed the stratification of patients $\geq$65 years into four risk groups, with a survival at 72 months of 0 for the highest risk group, 28% for the intermediate-high risk, 32% for the intermediate-low risk, and 69% for the lowest risk group.

3.3.3 Flow Cytometric Markers

The prognostic role of flow cytometric biomarkers in MM at diagnosis has not been clarified yet. In a prospective study by PETHEMA/GEM group evaluating the prognostic impact of several antigenic markers assessed by multiparameter flow cytometry (MFC) in transplant-eligible patients, the expression of both CD19 and CD28 as well as the absence of CD117 was associated with a significantly shorter PFS and OS [54]. Another Spanish prospective study [55] analyzed CD81 expression by MFC in myelomatous plasma cells from 230 MM patients included in the GEM05 > 65 years trial and detected the presence of CD81+ in approximately half of myeloma patients. CD81 expression was an independent prognostic factor for PFS (HR = 1.9; p = 0.003) and OS (HR = 2; p = 0.02). Particularly, elderly MM patients CD81+ had a median PFS of 21 months compared with 37 months in patients CD81- (p < 0.001), and a similar picture was observed for the 3-year OS in positive vs. negative CD81 patients (63% vs. 66%; p = 0.007). In a retrospective analysis of elderly patients enrolled in a phase III trial comparing VMPT-VT vs. VMP, a CD19+/CD117- bone marrow plasma cell immunophenotype was associated with a shorter OS but not a shorter PFS. By performing a separate analysis in the two therapeutic arms, this combination of antigens only had a negative impact in the VMP arm, suggesting a possible role of thalidomide in overcoming this adverse impact [40]. Finally, the number of clonal circulating plasma cells (cPCs) detected by MFC was found to be an independent prognostic factor in newly diagnosed MM patients treated with novel agents. In patients older than 65 years with a number of cPCs higher than 400, the median OS was 32 months, whereas it was not reached in those with cPSs less than 400 ($p = 0.021$) [56].

3.4 Response to Treatments and Minimal Residual Disease

In the new drug era, the achievement of the best response, which is a CR or even better, sCR has become an attainable goal in elderly MM patients [10, 14–16]. The impact of CR on long-term outcome observed in transplant-eligible MM patients [57, 58] was confirmed in elderly population receiving MP and novel agents [8]. A total of 1175 patients ≥65 years old were retrospectively analyzed to compare PFS and OS of CR patients receiving MP, MPT, VMP, or VMPT-VT with those whose best response was VGPR or PR. After a median follow-up of 29 months, patients who obtained the 3-year PFS were 67% in CR vs. 27% in VGPR patients (HR = 0.16; $p < 0.001$); the respective 3-year OS was 91% vs. 70% (HR 0.15; $p < 0.001$). Similar results were observed in patients older than 75 years. In multivariate analysis the achievement of a CR was the variable most strongly associated with significantly prolonged OS compared with VGPR (HR = 0.25; $p = 0.001$) and PR (HR = 0.16; $p < 0.001$). The addition of bortezomib or bortezomib plus thalidomide to MP was associated with longer OS as well, while the addition of thalidomide only was not. The significant increase in high-quality response rates obtained with novel agents has not been accompanied by the introduction of more sensitive methods for response assessment in clinical practice. The deeper level of response is currently defined by sCR requiring CR criteria plus normalization of free light chains ratio and the absence of clonal cells in bone marrow by immunohistochemistry and/or immunofluorescence [59]. However, recent studies suggest that immunophenotypic response assessed by MCF may represent a more accurate surrogate marker of outcome compared with conventional CR or sCR [60, 61]. This issue was confirmed in older patients included in the GEM05 > 65 years trial, receiving six induction cycles of VMP or VTP [62]. Immunophenotypic response after induction was detected in 30% of patients, and it translated into a significantly increased PFS and time to progression (TTP) compared with those in CR or sCR. In a multivariate Cox regression analysis for PFS, only immunophenotypic response after induction retained its prognostic value (RR 4.1; $p = 0.01$). A recent study [63] evaluated minimal residual disease (MRD) using an eight-color second-generation flow assay in 163 elderly MM patients randomized to nine VMP cycles followed by nine Rd cycles or to alternating cycles of VMP and Rd up to 18 cycles. Patients attaining MRD negativity at cycle nine showed a significantly prolonged TTP (median not reached vs. 35 months; $p = 0.001$) as compared to patients with persistent MRD. Similarly, the 3-year OS was 100% in patients MRD- and 72% in MRD+ patients ($p = 0.02$). Of note, the impact of attaining MRD negativity was irrespective of cytogenetic risk and age of patients.

3.5   Stratification by Host Factors

Age certainly still represents one of the main prognostic factors for survival in MM patients in the era of novel agents. A recent meta-analysis performed in 1435 patients with newly diagnosed MM treated with thalidomide- or bortezomib-based therapy demonstrated that patients aged 75 years or more had a significantly lower 3-year OS rate compared with younger subjects [64]. In addition, in a retrospective Greek analysis, octogenarians had significantly lower response rate, PFS, and OS and a higher 2-month mortality rate compared with patients aged 65 years or less [65]. Population-based studies suggest a marginal improvement in 10-year relative survival rate in patients aged more than 70 years also after the introduction of novel agents [3, 6, 66]. Nevertheless, older patients treated since 2010 seem to benefit more from latest therapeutic strategies as compared with younger subjects [67]. Subgroup analyses of the major, recent studies such as the VISTA [10, 43] and the FIRST trials [29, 30] or the MP vs. MPT meta-analysis [9] demonstrated that modern therapy was superior to the ancient one also in patients aged 75 years or more. On the contrary, in other trials such as MPR-R vs. MPR vs. MP [19] or VMP vs. VMPT-VP [15, 42], more intensive therapies did not show an advantage in older patients. A meta-analysis of four randomized trials including 1435 elderly patients with MM [64] demonstrated that age > 75 years, renal failure and developments of infections and cardiac and gastrointestinal complications leading to therapy discontinuation during the first 6 months of therapy were predictive of early mortality. This suggested the use of adapted therapy in those patients. Finally, high-dose melphalan followed by autotransplant has been successfully used for treating patients with MM aged 75 years and higher, although toxicity and mortality were higher [42, 68–70]. Although many elderly MM patients can tolerate such an intensive approach, at least one third of them experience severe adverse events leading to reduction and interruption of early treatment-related death. Defining which elderly patients may be able to tolerate and benefit from intensive therapy has been one of the main challenges in the MM research in the last few years.

The first attempt to build a frailty score and better define patients, beyond age, was made in a population-based MM registry study including 266 patients [71]. By performing univariate and multivariate analyses of classical prognostic factors of disease in conjunction with host factors such as age, performance status (PS), and comorbidity according to Charlson index, with therapy as a function of survival, only PS and comorbidity were in fact found to be related with OS in patients over 65 years. A "vulnerability score" was built using these variables: patients having both poor PS and high Charlson comorbidity index had a significantly shorter survival compared with those who had one or none of these adverse factors, regardless of therapy. That study allowed for the first time to distinguish between patients who could really benefit from effective therapy since their outcome depended on disease biology and patients whose outcome depended on host factors and thus for whom treatment should be tailored in order to minimize toxicity and mortality.

The Freiburg group conducted an analysis on 127 patients with MM aiming to develop a so-called Freiburg Comorbidity Index (FCI) based on Karnofsky PS and renal and lung disease status. This index was subsequently validated in an independent cohort of 466 patients, where it maintained its predictive roles in terms of survival. Together with ISS, this index allowed to stratify patients into low, intermediate, and high risk for mortality, consequently providing a valid guide to clinicians for personalized therapy [72]. The prognostic value of FCI on survival was recently confirmed by an Asian group in a retrospective study analyzing 127 elderly patients with MM [73].

However, PS often masked some geriatric impairment, and comorbidity did not completely explain the outcomes of elderly patients [74–76]. Therefore, a comprehensive geriatric assessment (CGA) including somatic, functional, and psychosocial domains was recommended before planning treatment for elderly cancer patients since 2005 [77]. Since then, this approach has been applied in several studies including patients with hematological malignancies. A recent systematic review of these relevant studies [78] showed that the majority of the domains considered in the geriatric assessment had a stronger predictive power for several clinical outcomes, mortality, toxicity, and therapy interruption as compared with age or PS. However, this study failed to draw any general recommendations on the best geriatric domains to use in clinical practice due to heterogeneity on patient populations, study designs, treatment regimens, types of geriatric assessment, and reported outcomes of selected studies. Moreover, a CGA is time consuming to be applied in everyday clinical practice. Therefore, in MM, a simplified geriatric assessment was chosen including patient's cognitive (Lawton's IADL: Instrumental Activities of Daily Living) and functional status and disability (Katz ADL: Activity Daily Living) [79]. These variables, together with age, PS, and comorbidity, were taken into consideration to build frailty scores.

Bila and coauthors [80] analyzed the effect of comorbidity according to Charlson index and IADL in 110 patients with MM aged more than 65 years. Patients with an age-adjusted CCI score ≥ 5 plus an IADL score < 3 had a significantly shorter survival; thus these parameters may be used to effectively personalize treatment.

However, the most comprehensive approach to frailty was proposed by the International Myeloma Working Group [81]. The IMWG evaluated 869 elderly MM patients included in three prospective trials [24, 31, 34] and analyzed age, PS, renal insufficiency, geriatric domains such as ADL and IADL, and Charlson comorbidity index (CCI) to provide a scoring system of frailty, predictive of clinical outcome and toxicity (Fig. 3.1). These variables were adjusted for ISS, cytogenetic, and therapy. That study found that age 75–80 and >80 years, CCI ≥ 2, ADL ≤ 4, and IADL ≤ 5 were significantly related to OS. Using the integer part of HR of these variables, a frailty score was calculated, and three groups of patients were identified: fit patients (39%, score 0), unfit patients (31%, score 1), and frail patients (30%, score ≥ 2). This frailty score was predictive for OS, PFS, cumulative incidence of non-hematological toxicity, and therapy discontinuation, whereas it was not for hematological toxicity. When this frailty score was adjusted for ISS stage, ISS retained its significance in each group of patients (fit, unfit, and frail) allowing to split patients in six categories with different OS (Table 3.1). Although this study has some limitations such as the retrospective design, the presence of patients

**Activities of Daily Living (ADL) and Instrumental Activities
of Daily Living (IADL)**

Score	ADL	IADL
0-1	Bathing (tub bath, shower, sponge bath)	Ability to use the telephone
0-1	Dressing (taking clothes from the wardrobe/drawers and getting dressed)	Shopping
0-1	Toileting (going to the toilet room, using toilet, arranging clothes)	Food preparation
0-1	Transferring	Housekeeping
0-1	Continence	Laundry
0-1	Feeding	Mode of transportation
0-1	–	Responsibility for own medications
0-1	–	Ability to handle finances

Charlson Comorbidity Index

Weight	Clinical condition
1	Myocardial infarction Congestive cardiac insufficiency Peripheral vascular disease Dementia Cerebrovascular disease Chronic pulmonary disease Conjunctive tissue disease Slight diabetes, without complications Ulcers Chronic diseases of the liver or cirrhosis
2	Hemiplegia Moderate or severe kidney disease Diabetes with complications Tumors Laukaemia Lymphoma
3	Moderate or severe liver disease
6	Malignant tumor, metastasis Aids

Fig. 3.1 Models Assessing Frailty in Multiple Myeloma

exclusively enrolled in trials, the absence of an external cohort useful for data validation, and the absence of a prospective validation study (that is ongoing), it is
today the best tool to personalize therapy in elderly patients with MM. How to
implement this tool in clinical practice remains to be defined.

Table 3.1 Frailty score adjusted for International Staging System

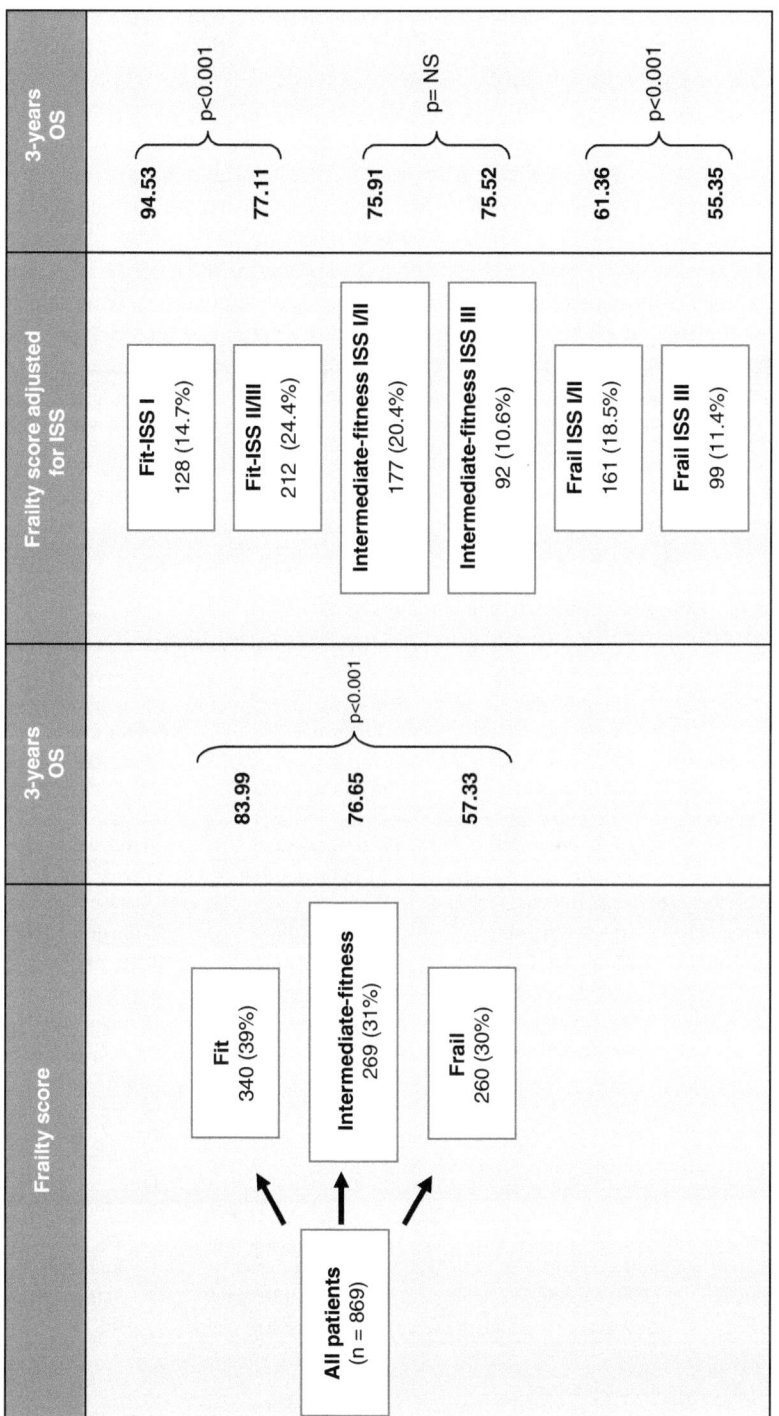

In addition, the frailty score can be calculated through the website www.myelo-mafrailtyscorecalculator.net allowing to know quickly the score of a patient and thus can be easily used in the daily clinical practice.

After appropriately stratifying patients and determining their prognosis, some crucial issues remain to be addressed. It has been suggested that this score should be used to adapt the dose of single drugs as described in Table 3.2. Nevertheless, two studies already demonstrated that high-dose dexamethasone is detrimental in elderly patients treated with thalidomide-dexamethasone [82] or lenalidomide-dexamethasone [83]. Moreover, peripheral neuropathy induced by bortezomib is not age or frailty dependent [84]. Once weekly and subcutaneously administration is now routinely used in clinical practice in elderly patients. Lenalidomide and melphalan, adjusted for renal function and blood count, are well tolerated also in very elderly patients since their hematological toxicity is not frailty dependent [81]. The major issue is not the single drugs per se or their dose but rather in which combinations the drug is used. Several studies demonstrated that two-drug combinations such as lenalidomide-dexamethasone or bortezomib-dexamethasone produce the same outcomes compared with three-drug combinations (adding alkylators or

Table 3.2 Dose adjustment according to frailty score

Prednisone	2 mg/kg day 1–4 of a 4–6 week cycles	1 mg/kg day 1–4 of a 4–6 week cycles	0.3 mg/kg day 1–4 of a 4–6 week cycles
	60 mg/m^2 day 1–4 of a 6 week cycle	300 mg/m^2 day 1–4 of a 6 week cycle	10 mg/m^2 day 1–4 of a 6 week cycle
Dexamethasone	40 mg day 1, 8, 15, 22 of a 28-day cycle	20 mg day 1, 8, 15, 22 of a 28-day cycle	10 mg day 1, 8, 15, 22 of a 28-day cycle
Melphalan	0.25 mg/kg day 1–4 of a 4–6 week cycle	0.18 mg/kg day 1–4 of a 4–6 week cycle	0.13 mg/kg day 1–4 of a 4–6 week cycle
	9 mg/m^2 day 1–4 of a 6 week cycle	7.5 mg/m^2 day 1–4 of a 6 week cycle	5 mg/m^2 day 1–4 of a 6 week cycle
Thalidomide	100–200 mg/day	50–100 mg/day	50 mg qod-50 mg/day
Lenalidomide	25 mg day 1–21 of a 28-day cycle	15 mg day 1–21 of a 28-day cycle	10 mg day 1–21 of a 28-day cycle
Bortezomib	1.3 mg/m^2 twice weekly day 1, 4, 8, 11 every 3 weeks	1.3 mg/m^2 once weekly day 1, 8, 15, 22 every 5 weeks	1.0 mg/m^2 once weekly day 1, 8, 15, 22 every 5 weeks

Table 3.3 Treatment algorithm for elderly MM patients

	Fit	Intermediate	Frail
Score	0	1	≥2
Dose	Full	Escalated[a]	Reduced
Treatment	Consider ASCT	Best available	Palliative care[b]
	Best available standard therapy	Standard therapy	Rd

[a]See text
[b]Preferable in high-risk patients

thalidomide) in elderly patient with MM [31, 32, 34]. Therefore, the frailty score should be considered also to select the most suitable regimen for each category of patients, as suggested in Table 3.3.

It is widely accepted that the treatment of fit patients may consist of intermediate-/high-dose melphalan followed by autologous stem cell transplantation in patients up to 70 years, or alternatively patients may receive the best available standard therapy in each country particularly in patients with ISS stages II–III (~25%) in whom the 3-year OS was at least 20% lower than that of patients with ISS stage I (95% vs. 77%, respectively).

Regarding frail patients, regimens containing adjusted dose of novel drugs or palliative therapy should be adopted. Further evidence is needed to choose which one of these two approaches should be used. Frail patients with high-risk disease by ISS stage (~10%) had the worst outcome (3-year OS = 55%, i.e., very similar to that obtained before novel drugs), and palliative therapy is a sensible strategy in these patients. On the contrary, in low-risk patients (~20%), disease control may be obtained through adapted doses of lenalidomide-dexamethasone, because this regimen showed to be very well tolerated also in older patients (FIRST) and may induce better results compared with palliative therapy. In this context, adequate and prompt supportive care to prevent infections, thromboembolism, and cardiac events is mandatory.

The real challenge is the selection of therapy in the intermediate-fitness group (or unfit) that represents approximately one third of patients. The 3-year OS and rate of discontinuation in unfit group (76% and 21%, respectively) seem to be closer to those of fit patients (84% and 16%, respectively) compared to those of frail ones (57% and 31%, respectively). Moreover, PFS and incidence of severe adverse events were not significantly different between unfit and fit patients. The dose intensity of novel agents that nearly 70% of intermediate-fitness patients were able to receive (80%) is closer to that fit patients rather than frail ones. There was no difference in terms of 3-year OS between unfit patients with ISS stages I–II and those with ISS stage III, and the forest plot for the risk of death comparing intermediate-fitness group and fit group by ISS, cytogenetic, therapy (bortezomib vs. lenalidomide), and regimen (doublet vs. triplet) did not show any significant difference among subgroups. In summary, in the intermediate-fitness group, the probability of undertreatment was much higher than the probability of overtreatment, as only less than one third of these patients are unsuitable to receive full-dose therapy. Such patients who are unsuitable for high-dose strategies are quite similar to frail subject. Nevertheless, there are no appropriate tools today to better distinguish them from intermediate-fitness patients who can tolerate full doses and who are more similar to fit patients. Thus, in the intermediate-fitness group, an approach with escalation of best available therapy combined with proper supportive care may be suitable. Further studies are urgently needed to minimize the size of the intermediate-fitness group.

Conclusions

The number of elderly patients with MM is expected to substantially increase in the next two decades. Novel agents now available and those under investigation have a remarkable potential to improve the outcome of elderly patients with MM. The chance to exploit this potential will mostly depend on how physicians will use these drugs.

Personalize therapy is clearly more and more needed, and it should be based no longer on age or PS only but on a more comprehensive evaluation of health, functional, and cognitive status of elderly patients. This is now possible by using frailty score as recommended by the IMWG. However, studies comparing different strategies in groups of defined by the frailty score are scant or lacking. We urgently need these studies to appropriately use the available regimens and those that will soon be approved. We also need to reduce the "intermediate" group, where uncertainty in outcome—and thus treatment—is still a concern. Biological markers of frailty may help us to have more robust predictive variables of toxicity useful for future precision medicine.

Biological characteristics and markers of tumor burden further help us to select therapy in some categories of elderly patients, although prospective studies in this field are lacking. Results of retrospective studies showed that, in elderly patients, no drug or combination is really able to overcome the poor prognosis associated with an unfavorable ISS stage, cytogenetic profile, or R-ISS stage.

As appropriate studies evaluating adjusted therapies are not available yet, physicians may adapt therapy according to suggestions of IMWG, by taking into account the specific treatment goals, as well as needs and preferences of patients.

Immunotherapy shows to be highly tolerated and effective; therefore it may represent the next step in the treatment of MM patients.

References

1. Smith BD, et al. Future of cancer incidence in the United States: burdens upon an aging, changing nation. J Clin Oncol. 2009;27:2758–65.
2. Turesson I, et al. Patterns of multiple myeloma during the past 5 decades: stable incidence rates for all ages groups in the population by rapidly changing age distribution in the clinic. Mayo Clinic Proc. 2010;85:225–30.
3. Brenner H, et al. Recent major improvement in long-term survival of younger patients with multiple myeloma. Blood. 2008;111:2521–6.
4. Kumar SK. Improved survival in multiple myeloma and the impact of novel therapies. Blood. 2008;111:2516–20.
5. Kumar S, Berdeja JG, Niesvizky R, et al. Long-term ixazomib maintenance is tolerable and improves depth of response following ixazomib-lenalidomide-dexamethasone induction in patients with previously untreated multiple myeloma: phase 2 study results. ASH Annual Meeting Abstracts 2014; abstract 82; 2013.
6. Schaapveld M, et al. Improved survival among younger but not among older patients with multiple myeloma in the Netherlands, a population-based study since 1989. Eur J Cancer. 2010;46:160–9.
7. Warren JL, et al. Multiple myeloma treatment transformed: a population-based study of changes in initial management approaches in the United States. J Clin Oncol. 2013;31:1984–9.
8. Gay F, et al. Complete response correlates with long-term progression-free and overall survival in elderly myeloma treated with novel agents: analysis of 1175 patients. Blood. 2011;117:3025–31.

9. Fayers PM, et al. Thalidomide for previously untreated elderly patients with multiple myeloma: meta-analysis of 1685 individual patients in six randomized clinical trials. Blood. 2011;118:1239–47.
10. San Miguel JF, et al. Bortezomib plus melphalan and prednisone for initial treatment of multiple myeloma. New Engl J Med. 2008;359:906–17.
11. Morabito F, et al. Bortezomib, melphalan, prednisone (VMP) versus melphalan, prednisone, thalidomide (MPT) in elderly newly diagnosed multiple myeloma patients: a retrospective case-matched study. Am J Hematol. 2014;89:355–62.
12. Moreau P, et al. Subcutaneous versus intravenous administration of bortezomib in patients with relapsed multiple myeloma: a randomised, phase 3, non-inferiority study. Lancet Oncol. 2011;12:431–40.
13. Bringhen S. Efficacy and safety of once-weekly bortezomib in multiple myeloma patients. Blood. 2010;116:4745–53.
14. Palumbo A, et al. Bortezomib as induction before autologous transplantation, followed by lenalidomide as consolidation-maintenance in untreated multiple myeloma patients. J Clin Oncol. 2010;28:800–7.
15. Palumbo A, et al. Bortezomib-melphalan-prednisone-thalidomide followed by maintenance with bortezomib-thalidomide compared with bortezomib-melphalan-prednisone for initial treatment of multiple myeloma: updated follow-up and improved survival. J Clin Oncol. 2014;32:634–40.
16. Mateos M-V, et al. Bortezomib, melphalan, and prednisone versus bortezomib, thalidomide, and prednisone as induction therapy followed by maintenance treatment with bortezomib and thalidomide versus bortezomib and prednisone in elderly patients with untreated multiple myeloma: a randomised trial. Lancet Oncol. 2010;11:934–41.
17. Mateos MV, et al. Sequential versus alternating administration of VMP and Rd in elderly patients with newly diagnosed MM. Blood. 2015;127(4):420–5.
18. Mateos MV, et al. An open-label, multicenter, phase 1b study of daratumumab in combination with pomalidomide-dexamethasone and with backbone regimens in patients with multiple myeloma. Haematologica 100 s1: abstract 275; 2015.
19. Palumbo A, et al. Continuous lenalidomide treatment for newly diagnosed multiple myeloma. N Engl J Med. 2012;366:1759–69.
20. Zweegman S, et al. Melphalan, prednisone, and lenalidomide versus melphalan, prednisone, and thalidomide in untreated multiple myeloma. Blood. 2016;127:1109–16.
21. Stewart AK, et al. Melphalan, prednisone, and thalidomide vs melphalan, prednisone, and lenalidomide (ECOG E1A06) in untreated multiple myeloma. Blood. 2015;126:1294–301.
22. O'Donnell E, et al. A phase II study of modified lenalidomide, bortezomib, and dexamethasone (RVD lite) for transplant-ineligible patients with newly diagnosed multiple myeloma. ASH Annual Meeting Abstracts: abstract 3454; 2014.
23. Moreau P, et al. Phase 1/2 study of carfilzomib plus melphalan and prednisone in patients aged over 65 years with newly diagnosed multiple myeloma. Blood. 2015;125:3100–4.
24. Bringhen S, et al. Carfilzomib, cyclophosphamide and dexamethasone in patients with newly diagnosed multiple myeloma: a multicenter, phase 2 study. Blood. 2014;124:63–9.
25. Bringhen S, et al. Weekly carfilzomib, cyclophosphamide and dexamethasone (wCCyd) in elderly newly diagnosed multiple myeloma patients: results of a phase 2 study. ASH Annual Meeting Abstracts: abstract 1828; 2015.
26. Dytfeld D, et al. Carfilzomib, lenalidomide and low-dose dexamethasone in elderly patients with newly diagnosed multiple myeloma. Haematologica. 2014;99:162–4.
27. Kumar SK, et al. Safety and tolerability of ixazomib, an oral proteasome inhibitor, in combination with lenalidomide and dexamethasone in patients with previously untreated multiple myeloma: an open-label phase 1/2 study. Lancet Oncol. 2014;15:1503–12.
28. Dimopoulos MA, et al. Randomized phase 2 study of the all-oral combination of investigational proteasome inhibitor ixazomib plus cyclophosphamide and low-dose dexamethasone (ICd) in patients with newly diagnosed multiple myeloma who are transplant-ineligible. ASH Annual Meeting Abstracts: abstract 26; 2015.

29. Benboubker L, et al. Lenalidomide and dexamethasone in transplant-ineligible patients with myeloma. N Engl J Med. 2014;371:906–17.
30. Hulin C, et al. Update outcomes and impact of age with lenalidomide and low-dose dexamethasone or melphalan, prednisone, and thalidomide in randomized, phase III FIRST Trial. J Clin Oncol. 2016;34:3609–17.
31. Magarotto V, et al. Triplet vs doublet lenalidomide-containing regimens for the treatment of elderly patients with newly diagnosed multiple myeloma. Blood. 2016;127:1102–8.
32. Niesvizky R, et al. Community-based phase IIIB trial of three UPFRONT bortezomib-based myeloma regimens. J Clin Oncol. 2015;33:3921–9.
33. Falco P, et al. Lenalidomide-prednisone induction followed by lenalidomide-melphalan-prednisone consolidation and lenalidomide-prednisone maintenance in newly diagnosed elderly unfit myeloma patients. Leukemia. 2013;27:695–701.
34. Larocca A, et al. A phase 2 study of three low-dose intensity subcutaneous bortezomib regimens in elderly frail patients with untreated multiple myeloma. Leukemia. 2016;30:1320–26.
35. Avet-Loiseau H, et al. Genetic abnormalities and survival in multiple myeloma: the experience of the Intergroupe Francophone du Myelome. Blood. 2007;109:3489–95.
36. Gertz MA, et al. Clinical implications of t(11;14)(q13; q32), t(4 ;14)(p16.3;q32), and -17p13 in myeloma patients treated with high-dose therapy. Blood. 2005;106:2837–40.
37. Usmani SZ, et al. Defining and treating high-risk multiple myeloma. Blood. 2015;29:2119–25.
38. Nilsson T, et al. A pooled analysis of karyotypic patterns, breakpoints and imbalances in 783 cytogenetically abnormal multiple myeloma reveals frequently involved chromosome segments as well as significant age- and sex-related differences. Br J Haematol. 2003;120:960–9.
39. Avet-Loiseau H, et al. Chromosomal abnormalities are major prognostic factors in elderly patients with multiple myeloma: the Intergroupe Francophone du Myelome experience. J Clin Oncol. 2013;31:2806–9.
40. Caltagirone S, et al. Chromosome 1 abnormalities in elderly patients with newly diagnosed multiple myeloma treated with novel therapies. Haematologica. 2014;99:1611–7.
41. Morgan GJ, et al. Long-term follow-up of MRC myeloma IX trial: survival outcomes with bisphosphonate and thalidomide treatment. Clin Cancer Res. 2013;19:6030–8.
42. Palumbo A, et al. Bortezomib-melphalan-prednisone-thalidomide followed by maintenance with bortezomib-thalidomide compared with bortezomib-melphalan-prednisone for initial treatment of multiple myeloma: a randomized controlled trial. J Clin Oncol. 2010;34:5101–8.
43. Mateos MV, et al. Bortezomib plus melphalan and prednisone compared with melphalan and prednisone in previously untreated multiple myeloma: updated follow-up and impact of subsequent therapy in the phase III VISTA trial. J Clin Oncol. 2010;28:2259–66.
44. Mateos MV, et al. Outcome according to cytogenetic abnormalities and DNA ploidy in myeloma patients receiving short induction with weekly bortezomib followed by maintenance. Blood. 2011;118:4547–53.
45. Avet-Loiseau H, et al. Impact of cytogenetics on outcome of transplant-ineligible patients with newly diagnosed multiple myeloma treated with continuous lenalidomide plus low-dose dexamethasone in the First (MM-020) Trial. ASH Annual Meeting Abstracts: abstract 730; 2015.
46. Vu T, et al. Characteristics of exceptional responders to lenalidomide-based therapy in multiple myeloma. Blood Cancer J. 2015;5:e363.
47. Kumar S, et al. Trisomies in multiple myeloma: impact on survival in patients with high-risk cytogenetics. Blood. 2012;119:2100–5.
48. Greipp PR, et al. International staging system for multiple myeloma. J Clin Oncol. 2005;23:3412–2320.
49. Avet-Loiseau H, et al. Combining fluorescent in situ hybridization data with ISS staging improves risk assessment in myeloma: an International Myeloma Working Group collaborative project. Leukemia. 2013;27:711–7.
50. Palumbo A, et al. Revised International Staging System for multiple myeloma: a report from International Myeloma Working Group. J Clin Oncol. 2015;33:2863–69.
51. Shaughnessy JD, et al. A validates gene expression model of high-risk multiple myeloma is defined by deregulated expression of genes mapping to chromosome 1. Blood. 2007;109:2276–84.

52. Kuiper R, et al. A gene expression signature for high-risk multiple myeloma. Leukemia. 2012;26:2406–13.
53. Kuiper R, et al. Prediction of high- and low-risk multiple myeloma based on gene expression and the International Staging System. Blood. 2015;126:1996–2004.
54. Mateo G, et al. Prognostic value of immunophenotyping in multiple myeloma: a study by the PETHEMA/GEM cooperative study groups on patients uniformly treated with high-dose therapy. J Clin Oncol. 2008;26:2737–44.
55. Paiva B, et al. Clinical significance of CD81 expression by clonal plasma cells in high-risk smoldering and symptomatic multiple myeloma patients. Leukemia. 2012;26:1862–9.
56. Gonsalves MI, et al. Quantification of clonal circulating plasma cells in newly diagnosed multiple myeloma: implications for redefining high-risk myeloma. Leukemia. 2014;28:2060–5.
57. Cavo M, et al. Bortezomib with thalidomide plus dexamethasone compared with thalidomide plus dexamethasone as induction therapy before, and consolidation therapy after double autologous stem-cell transplantation in newly diagnosed multiple myeloma: a randomized phase 3 study. Lancet. 2010;376:2075–85.
58. Kapoor P, et al. Importance of achieving stringent complete response after autologous stem-cell transplantation in multiple myeloma. J Clin Oncol. 2013;31:4529–35.
59. Durie BG, et al. International uniform response criteria for multiple myeloma. Leukemia. 2006;20:1467–73.
60. Martinez-Lopez J, et al. Critical analysis of the stringent complete response in multiple myeloma: contribution of sFLC and bone marrow clonality. Blood. 2015;126:858–62.
61. Rawstron AC, et al. Minimal residual disease assessed by multiparameter flow cytometry in multiple myeloma: impact on outcome in the Medical Research Council Myeloma IX study. J Clin Oncol. 2013;31:2540–7.
62. Paiva B, et al. Comparison of immunofixation, serum free light chain, and immunophenotyping for response evaluation and prognostication in multiple myeloma. Blood. 2011;29:1627–33.
63. Paiva B, et al. The relevance of minimal residual disease (MRD) monitoring in elderly multiple myeloma patients. ASH Annual Meeting Abstracts: abstract 4181; 2015.
64. Bringhen S, et al. Age and organ damage correlate with poor survival in myeloma patients: meta-analysis of 1435 individual patient data from 4 randomized trials. Haematologica. 2013;98:980–7.
65. Dimopoulos MA, et al. Myeloma in octogenarians: disease characteristics and clinical outcomes in the era of modern anti-myeloma therapy. ASH Annual Meeting Abstracts: abstract 4738; 2014.
66. Pulte D, et al. Improvement in survival of older adults with multiple myeloma: results of an updated period analysis of SEER data. Oncologist. 2011;16:1600–3.
67. Kumar SK, et al. Continued improvement in survival in multiple myeloma: changes in early mortality and outcomes in older patients. Leukemia. 2014;28:1122–8.
68. Badros A, et al. Autologous stem cell transplantation in elderly multiple myeloma patients over the age of 70 years. Br J Haematol. 2001;114:600–7.
69. Facon T, et al. Melphalan and prednisone plus thalidomide versus melphalan and prednisone alone or reduced-intensity autologous stem cell transplantation in elderly patients with multiple myeloma (IFM 99–06): a randomised trial. Lancet. 2007;370:1209–18.
70. Palumbo A, et al. Dose-intensive melphalan with stem cell support (MEL100) is superior to standard treatment in elderly myeloma patients. Blood. 1999;94:1248–53.
71. Offidani M, et al. Assessment of vulnerability measures and their effect on survival in a real-life population of multiple myeloma patients registered at Marche Region multiple myeloma registry. Clin Lymphoma Myeloma Leuk. 2012;12:423–32.
72. Kleber M, et al. Validation of the Freiburg Comorbidity Index in 466 multiple myeloma patients and combination with the international staging system are highly predictive for outcome. Clin Lymphoma Myeloma Leuk. 2013;13:541–51.
73. Kim SM, et al. Comparison of the Freiburg and Charlson comorbidity indices in predicting overall survival in elderly patients with newly diagnosed multiple myeloma. Biomed Res Int. 2014;2014:437852.

74. Corsetti MT, et al. Hematologic improvement and response in elderly AML/RAEB patients treated with valproic acid and low-dose Ara-C. Leuk Res. 2011;35:991–7.
75. Klepin HD, et al. The feasibility of inpatient geriatric assessment for older adult receiving induction chemotherapy for acute myelogenous leukemia. J Am Geriatr Soc. 2011;59:1837–46.
76. Muffly LS, et al. Pilot study of comprehensive geriatric assessment (CGA) in allogeneic transplant: CGA captures a high prevalence of vulnerabilities in older transplant recipients. Biol Blood Marrow Transplant. 2013;19:429–34.
77. Extermann M, et al. Use of comprehensive geriatric assessment in older cancer patients: recommendations from the task force on CGA of the International Society of Geriatric Oncology (SIOG). Crit Rev Oncol Hematol. 2005;55:241–52.
78. Haymaker ME, et al. The relevance of a geriatric assessment for elderly patients with a haematological malignancy—a systematic review. Leuk Res. 2014;38:275–83.
79. Lawton MP. Scales to measure competence in everyday activities. Phychopharmacol Bull. 1988;24:609–14.
80. Bila J, et al. Prognostic effect of comorbidity indices in elderly patients with multiple myeloma. Clin Lymphoma Myeloma Leuk. 2015;15:416–9.
81. Palumbo A, et al. Geriatric assessment predicts survival and toxicities in elderly myeloma patients: an International Myeloma Working Group report. Blood. 2015;125:2068–74.
82. Ludwig H, et al. Thalidomide-dexamethasone compared to melphalan-prednisolone in elderly patients with multiple myeloma. Blood. 2009;113:3435–42.
83. Rajkumar SV, et al. Lenalidomide plus high-dose dexamethasone versus lenalidomide plus low-dose dexamethasone as initial therapy for newly diagnosed multiple myeloma: an open-label randomised controlled trial. Lancet Oncol. 2010;11:29–37.
84. Delforge M, et al. Treatment-related peripheral neuropathy in multiple myeloma: the challenge continues. Lancet Oncol. 2010;11:1086–95.

Treatment of t(4;14) and del(17p) in Multiple Myeloma

4

Pieter Sonneveld

4.1   Introduction

Multiple myeloma (MM) is a proliferation of monoclonal plasma cells which produce a monoclonal protein [1]. In general indications for treatment are based on the presence of organ damage, specifically hypercalcemia, renal impairment, anemia, or lytic bone lesions. More recently markers of active disease were identified that indicate a need for treatment, i.e., an involved/uninvolved serum free light chain ratio ≥ 100, bone marrow plasma cells $\geq 60\%$, or >1 lesion on MRI [2].

MM is associated with chromosomal instability, and cytogenetic abnormalities (CA) may have a critical impact on prognosis [1–4]. Response to treatment and survival of newly diagnosed MM (NDMM) varies from 2 to >10 years, depending on risk factors, age, transplant eligibility, and access to treatment. In this chapter we will discuss the biological background and potential impact of high-risk (HR) CA, specifically t(4;14) and del(17p), and provide recommendations for treatment of these high-risk NDMM patients. Parts of this chapter were previously published in a consensus guideline of the International Myeloma Working Group [5].

This chapter was partly published before as: Sonneveld P, Avet-Loiseau H, Lonial S, Usmani S, Siegel D, Anderson KC, Chng WJ, Moreau P, Attal M, Kyle RA, Caers J, Hillengass J, San Miguel J, van de Donk NW, Einsele H, Bladé J, Durie BG, Goldschmidt H, Mateos MV, Palumbo A, Orlowski R. Treatment of multiple myeloma with high-risk cytogenetics: a consensus of the International Myeloma Working Group. Blood. 2016 Jun 16;127(24):2955–62. doi: 10.1182/blood-2016-01-631200. Epub 2016 Mar 21. PMID:27002115.

P. Sonneveld, M.D., Ph.D.
Department of Hematology, Erasmus MC Cancer Institute, Erasmus MC,
Rm Na822, PO Box 2040, 3000 Rotterdam, The Netherlands
e-mail: p.sonneveld@erasmusmc.nl

© Springer International Publishing AG 2018
S.Z. Usmani, A.K. Nooka (eds.), *Personalized Therapy for Multiple Myeloma*,
https://doi.org/10.1007/978-3-319-61872-2_4

4.2 Diagnostic Procedures to Detect t(4;14) and del(17p)

4.2.1 Conventional Karyotyping

Conventional karyotyping is performed on metaphase cells. Unlike acute leukemia, the majority of myeloma plasma cells do not proliferate. Therefore, this technique reveals CA in only 20–30% of patients, the majority of which are numerical abnormalities. Several translocations including t(4;14) cannot be detected by this technique. The normal karyotype in patients with a low proliferation index corresponds to the kinetics of normal bone marrow cells, while plasma cells usually have a low proliferation. However, when an abnormal karyotype is detected, it has an unfavorable impact as was demonstrated for del(13q) [6]. Since more sensitive techniques have become available such as interphase fluorescence in situ hybridization (FISH) and single-nucleotide polymorphisms (SNP) arrays that detect CA in nearly all MM, karyotyping is no longer a routine test.

4.2.2 Fluorescence In Situ Hybridization (FISH)

FISH is performed in interphase cells, thereby overcoming the problem of low tumor cell proliferation rate in classical karyotyping. Pretest purification of CD138 expressing plasma cells is required, or dual staining for cytoplasmic Ig and FISH should be performed. Currently FISH is the standard technique for analysis of CA in myeloma. Samples are usually screened for CA, which occur in >1% of patients. FISH is a practical cytogenetic tool to detect t(4;14) and del(17p) for routine diagnosis. It does not detect single-nucleotide variants [7]. TP53 on chromosome 17p is deleted in 7% of myeloma, yet mutated at a much higher frequency based on exome sequencing. Knowing these restrictions, FISH testing in clinical trials may include gain(1q), del(1p), t(4;14)(p16;q32), t(14;16)(q32;q23), del(17p13), and a marker for aneuploidy (Table 4.1). For routine diagnostic testing, t(4;14) and del(17p13) suffice.

4.2.3 Single-Nucleotide Polymorphisms (SNP)-Based Mapping Arrays

High-resolution genome-wide analysis of single-nucleotide polymorphisms detects regions with loss of heterozygosity and numerical abnormalities. SNP mapping arrays identify copy number variations (CNVs) [8]. Translocations are not routinely detected and will require additional FISH.

4.2.4 Comparative Genomic Hybridization (CGH)

Array-based comparative genomic hybridization (aCGH) is a tool for genome-wide classification of CNVs, which primarily detects numerical abnormalities. Using

Table 4.1 Primary and secondary genetic events that can be identified by FISH

Primary genetic events			Secondary genetic events		
IgH translocation	Gene(s)	Frequency (%)	Deletion	Gene(s)	Frequency (%)
t(4;14)	*FGFR3/MMSET*	15	1p	*CDKN2C, FAF1, FAM46C*	30
t(6;14)	*CCND3*	4	6q		33
t(11;14)	*CCND1*	20	8p		25
t(14;16)	*MAF*	4	13	*RB1, DIS3*	44
t(14;20)	*MAFB*	1	11q	*BIRC2/BIRC3*	7
			14q	*TRAF3*	38
			16q	*WWOX, CYLD*	35
			17p	*TP53*	7
Hyperdiploidy			**Gain**		
Trisomies of chromosomes 3, 5, 7, 9, 11, 15, 19, 21	NA	50	1q	*CKS1B, ANP32E*	40

CGH or SNP arrays, chromosomal changes can be observed in 90% of myeloma patients [9].

4.2.5 Gene Expression Profiling (GEP)

GEP is a technique to identify expression of genes and pathways. Based on RNA expression using microarrays, subgroups of patients are identified with a unique GEP phenotype which partly corresponds to the TC classification [10]. GEP can be used to identify high-risk profiles with significant prognostic significance [11].

4.3 High-Risk CA

4.3.1 IgH Translocations: t(4;14)

MM chromosome translocations involving the immunoglobulin heavy chain (IgH) locus on chromosome 14 and hyperdiploidy with multiple copies of odd-numbered chromosomes are considered primary events (Table 4.1) [12]. IgH translocations are observed in 40% of patients. Frequently involved partner chromosomes/loci for the IgH locus are 4p16 (*FGFR3/MMSET*) (12–15%), 11q13 (*CCND1*) (15–20%), 16q23 (*MAF*) (3%), 6p21 (*CCND3*) (<5%), and 20q11 (*MAFB*) (1%) [13].

Translocation (4;14) involves the IgH locus (14q32) and leads to a deregulation of fibroblast growth factor receptor 3 (*FGFR3*) and the multiple myeloma *SET* domain (*MMSET*) [14–16]. This translocation is considered a primary or initiating oncogenic event, and it is mutually exclusive with other translocations.

MMSET is a chromatin remodeling factor and overexpressed in all tumors with this translocation. It may have DNA repair functions and posttranscriptionally enhances MYC. FGFR3 contributes to B-cell oncogenesis, but its role in the pathogenesis of MM has not been elaborated. Since *FGFR3* is not expressed in one third of patients with t(4;14), the target gene is most likely *MMSET*.

t(4;14) is associated with impaired PFS/OS in many trials [9]. As will be discussed later, bortezomib may at least partly improve the negative prognostic impact of t(4;14) [17–20]. Prolonged survival was reported in t(4;14) treated with high-dose therapy (HDT) and tandem autologous transplant (ASCT) [21, 22]. SNP arrays have showed that the adverse impact of t(4;14) is heterogenous and may be related to the presence of concomitant CA [23].

4.3.2 Genomic Imbalance: del(17p) and Other Deletions or Additions

Hyperdiploidy occurs in more than half of NDMM patients and is associated with improved PFS/OS [14, 24]. In the MRC IX trial, coexisting hyperdiploidy did not abrogate the poor prognosis of adverse CA [25]. In contrast, in a retrospective analysis, PFS of patients with t(4;14) was negatively impacted by del(1p32), del22q, and >30 structural CA, while del(6q) worsened PFS and del(1p32) worsened OS and >8 numerical changes improved OS in del(17p) [23]. Modern techniques such as SNP arrays identify significantly more CNVs above karyotypic hyperdiploidy [26].

Deletions of the TP53 locus occur in 8–10% of newly diagnosed MM, and the incidence increases with disease progression [27]. TP53 mutations are much more frequent in patients with del(17p) deletions than in patients without these. It is uncertain if the adverse prognostic impact of del(17p) is due to haploinsufficiency or complete inactivation of TP53. Deletion of *TP53* induces clonal immortalization and survival of (myeloma) tumor cells [28].

At present it is not clear which minimum percentage of cells carrying del(17p) nor the CA load of other genetic imbalances is required for an adverse prognosis nor whether this varies with the choice of therapy and stage of disease. Minimal percentages of 20 and 60% have been recommended for del(17p) [15, 23].

The prognostic impact of CA may vary from diagnosis to (refractory) disease due to the selection of disease subclones which may have different CA in various stages of the disease [29]. In solitary plasmacytoma or extramedullary disease, del(17p) may occur even more frequently [30, 31].

4.3.3 Multiple Adverse CA

Among patients with an adverse IgH translocation, 62% have concomitant gain(1q), compared to 32.4% in controls [15]. The frequency of del(17p) is similar in patients with or without adverse IgH translocations. Among patients with an IgH translocation and/or gain1q or del(17p), 20% share 2 or more CA. When CA occur in isolation, each lesion had a similar impact on OS. The triple combination of an adverse IgH translocation, gain(1q), and del(17p) has been associated with a median OS of only 9.1 months demonstrating the progressive impact of combined multiple adverse CA on OS [15]. The French IFM group showed that of 110 patients displaying either t(4;14) or del(17p), in 25 both CA were present. In patients with t(4;14), PFS was worse in case of concomitant presence of del(1p32), del(22q), and/or >30 structural changes. In patients with del(17p), del(6q) further reduced PFS, whereas the presence of gain15 and del14 had a protective effect [23].

4.3.4 Good Combined with Adverse CA

In the Myeloma IX study, 58% of patients had hyperdiploidy [32]. Of these, 61% had one or more adverse lesions (t(4;14), t(14;16), t(14;20), gain1q, or del(17p)). OS and PFS were worse in patients with hyperdiploidy plus an adverse lesion, compared to hyperdiploidy alone (median PFS 23 vs. 15.4 months; median OS 60.9 vs. 35.7 months).

Finally, in a large analysis, the presence of trisomies reduced the adverse impact of t(4;14), t(14;16), t(14;20), or *TP53* deletion in patients with MM [33].

4.4 Cytogenetic Risk Classifications

The definition of high-risk disease is subject to diagnostic and treatment options. With median PFS and OS of transplant-eligible (TE) patients approaching 4 and 10 years, most investigators consider HR disease as OS <3 years, with ultra-HR disease having a survival <2 years. For nontransplant-eligible patients (NTE) OS <2 years is considered HR [34, 35]. It is important to define HR disease based on objective criteria (Table 4.2).

4.4.1 Risk Classifications Based on FISH

The International Myeloma Working Group (IMWG) proposed a model of HR MM defined as at least one of the following: del17p, t(4;14), or t(14;16) determined by FISH [27]. The Mayo Clinic classification added hypodiploidy and t(14;20) for the definition of HR MM [36]. Later classifications attempted to separate MM into several risk groups. In MRC IX, three groups were identified, i.e., favorable risk (no adverse IgH translocation, del(17p), or gain(1q)), intermediate risk (one adverse

Table 4.2 Summary of cytogenetic risk features

	High risk	Standard risk
Cytogenetic abnormality	FISH: t(4;14), t(14;16), t(14;20), del(17/17p), gain(1q) Non-hyperdiploid karyotype, karyotype del(13) GEP: high-risk signature	All others including: FISH: t(11;14), t(6;14)

CA), and high risk (>1 adverse CA). Median PFS/OS of patients with FR, IR, or HR was 23.5, 17.8, and 11.7 months and 60.6, 41.9, and 21.7 months, respectively [15]. Ultrahigh risk was defined as three or more CA (2%, median OS 9 months). These classifications were defined when access to novel drugs was still limited and may change when additional treatment modalities are becoming available. An example is t(4;14) which may be IR rather than HR when novel agents are given [17, 37–39].

4.4.2 Risk Classifications Based on FISH and ISS

The combination of ISS with high-risk CA reflects tumor mass, patient condition, and genetics. The IMWG showed that t(4;14) and/or del(17p) separates two groups with different EFS and OS within each ISS stage [40]. Combining t(4;14) and del(17p) with ISS stage improved prognostic staging [40]. Neben et al. combined ISS with t(4;14) or del(17p) [14]. Using this stratification median, PFS after ASCT was 2.7, 2.0, and 1.2 years for the FR group (ISS I, no HR CA), IR(ISS I and HR CA or ISS II/III without HR CA), and HR (ISS II/III and HR CA), respectively. Five-year OS were 72%, 62%, and 41%, respectively. Identical results were obtained in the HOVON65/GMMG-HD4 trial [41].

The MRC IX study combined ISS and the presence of 0, 1, or >1 adverse CA. Median OS in the ultra-HR group, defined by ISS II or III plus >1 adverse CA, were 9.9 and 19.4 months, compared with OS 67.8 months in the favorable group [15].

4.4.3 Risk Classifications Based on FISH, ISS, and LDH

A meta-analysis of randomized trials in NDMM confirmed that combining ISS, serum lactodehydrogenase (LDH), and FISH identifies four risk groups including a very high-risk population (5–8%). Patients with ISS stage III, elevated LDH, and t(4;14) or del(17p) have a 2-year OS of only 54.6% [42]. More recently the revised ISS was defined, incorporating HR FISH (t(4;14), t(14;16), del(17p)) with ISS and LDH [43].

4.4.4 Gene Expression Profiling (GEP)

The prognostic impact of GEP by microarray was examined in several studies. The UAMS identified a 70-gene subset as an independent prognosticator [44]. The presence of a HR signature (13.1%) resulted in inferior EFS (5-year EFS, 18% vs. 60%) and OS (5-year OS, 28% vs. 78%). In this signature, several genes mapped to chromosome 1(q) and (1p) [22]. The same group performed GEP analysis 48 h after bortezomib dosing in TT3 [45]. Based on GEP changes, the UAMS-80 signature was constructed.

The EMC-92 signature was derived from patients in the HOVON65/GMMG-HD4 trial. When combined with ISS, it predicts impaired PFS and OS across treatments [46, 47]. OS of HR patients (21%) at 5 years was 10% as compared with 72% for others (79%). Other GEP-based risk models include the IFM-15 and MRC-IX-6 gene signatures [48]. In general, these GEP signatures are useful for prognostication while prediction has to be validated. There is no complete concordance with FISH abnormalities [49].

4.4.5   mSMART

The Mayo Stratification of Myeloma and Risk-Adapted Therapy (mSMART) criteria use a combination of FISH, plasma cell labeling index (PCLI), and GEP as tools to identify three risk categories (SR, IR, HR) for prognostication of patients with NDMM [50]. In mSMART del(17p) and t(4;14) are included as high-risk and intermediate-risk factors, respectively. Patients can be stratified for different therapeutic approaches [39]. However, risk-adapted therapy has not been validated in prospective studies.

4.5   Treatment Options with Novel Agents for High-Risk Disease Characterized by t(4;14) and/or del(17p)

The International Myeloma Working Group (IMWG) recommends to use the combination of FISH, LDH, and ISS stage for risk stratification in NDMM [39]. Other features such as renal failure, plasma cell proliferative rate, and presence of extramedullary disease also contribute to risk. GEP is emerging as a prognostic tool for risk stratification.

Recently two reviews addressed the issue of general treatment strategies for HR myeloma [51, 52]. Here we address the treatment choices for patients with HR NDMM based on cytogenetic profile with for t(4;14) and/or del(17/17p).

4.5.1   Thalidomide

Thalidomide does not overcome the adverse impact of high-risk CA in MM. In the UAMS trial for RRMM, del(13q) by karyotyping had a shorter survival with thalidomide [53]. Three trials studying thalidomide during induction in NDMM (MRC IX: CTD vs. CTDa; HOVON50/GMMG-HD2: VAD vs. TAD; GEM2005:TD) observed shorter OS in HR CA [54–57]. Thalidomide maintenance did not improve survival in HR CA in three trials: MRC IX (3-year OS 45% vs. 69%), HOVON50 (3-year OS 17% vs. 69%) trials, and Total Therapy 2 (TT2, 5-year OS 56% vs. 72%) [17, 20, 24, 54, 55, 58]. In MRC IX 3-year OS was worse in patients with HR-CA (45%) [59]. In HOVON50/GMMG-HD2 PFS1 was better with thalidomide treatment, but second PFS was significantly shorter, resulting in a reduced OS [57]. In

TT2 the presence of CA was associated with inferior survival, and a benefit with thalidomide was only observed in a subgroup of patients after 10 years [60].

From these data it can be concluded that thalidomide does not abrogate the adverse effect of t(4;14) and del(17) CA in transplant-eligible patients. Conclusive data for elderly or frail patients are not available.

4.5.2 Bortezomib

Several randomized trials have evaluated bortezomib for induction, consolidation, or maintenance treatment in cytogenetic subgroups. In IFM-2005-01 bortezomib/dexamethasone showed a superior response and OS compared with VAD. This combination resulted in a better EFS and OS for patients with t(4;14) but did not improve outcome in del(17p) (4-year OS 50% vs. 79%) [61]. In HOVON65/GMMG-HD4 bortezomib-based induction and maintenance showed an improved outcome for patients with del(17p) (median PFS 26 vs. 12 months);(3-year OS, 69% vs. 17%)). At long-term follow-up, this advantage is still present. However, OS remains inferior to patients without del(17p) (3-year OS, 85%). In patients with t(4;14), PFS was not better with bortezomib (25 vs. 22 months), while OS was improved (3-year OS 69% vs. 44%) compared with 85% in patients without t(4;14) [41]. In the GEM 2005 trial, VTD followed by ASCT and maintenance did not improve OS in HR CA (3-year OS, 60% vs. 88%) [56]. The GIMEMA group compared VTD with TD for induction and consolidation with double ASCT. In the subgroup of 25% with t(4;14), OS was 69% vs. 37% in favor of VTD as compared with 74% vs. 63% without t(4;14) and/or del(17p) [19]. A meta-analysis of four randomized trials showed that the odds of posttransplantation CR + nCR in bortezomib-treated patients were similar for high-risk (del(17p) + t(4;14)) and SR (2.44 vs. 1.67, n.s.) cytogenetics [18]. These trials (1874 patients) showed that bortezomib plus ASCT was superior (PFS 41 vs. 33 months) ($p < 0.0001$). In patients with HR FISH, this was 32 vs. 22 months ($p < 0.0001$). PFS benefit was observed in patients with t(4;14) but lacking del(17p) (36 vs. 24 months, $p = 0.001$) and in del(17p) lacking t(4;14) (27 vs. 19 months, $p = 0.014$), but not in patients carrying both CA [62]. In TT3 OS was significantly shorter in patients with a HR profile (2-year OS 56% vs. 88%) compared with SR GEP profile, with exception of low TP53 expression [63]. Addition of bortezomib improved OS compared with TT2 in LR MM [63, 64].

Data in NTE patients are scarce. The VISTA trial combined melphalan/prednisone with bortezomib (VMP vs. MP). In patients treated with VMP, HR-CA did not influence outcome when compared with SR (OS, 56% vs. 71%) [65]. In a Pethema trial comparing VMP with VPT (bortezomib/thalidomide/prednisone) followed by maintenance with VT vs. VP, HR patients had shorter PFS than SR patients from the first (24 vs. 33 months) and second randomization (17 vs. 27 months) and shorter survival (3-year OS, 55% vs. 77%) [66]. The GIMEMA group compared VMP with VMPT. In this bortezomib-dense treatment, HR vs. SR patients had similar PFS [67]. The IFM group observed that across bortezomib regimens, no benefit was achieved in HR-CA NTE patients [68]. From these data it can be concluded that bortezomib partly overcomes the adverse effect of t(4;14) and possibly del(17p) on CR, PFS, and OS. There is no benefit in t(4;14) combined with del(17p) in transplant-eligible patients. In transplant-ineligible patients, VMP may partly restore PFS in high-risk cytogenetics, although data are scarce.

4.5.3   Novel IMiDs: Lenalidomide and Pomalidomide

Experience with lenalidomide in first-line therapy for HR-CA patients is limited. In HR-CA PFS with lenalidomide was inferior as compared with SR patients (18 vs. 26 months) [69]. In the GIMEMA trial comparing high-dose melphalan with MPR, there was a trend for better PFS with lenalidomide maintenance in SR as compared with HR-CA (HR 0.38 (0.24–0.62) vs. 0.73 (0.37–1.42)). However, there was no effect on OS [70]. In the IFM 2005-02 trial, lenalidomide maintenance did not overcome the poor prognosis of t(4;14) (27 vs. 24 months) and only partly of del(17p) (29 vs. 14 months vs. 42 months in all patients) [71]. Convincing data for continuous lenalidomide in CA groups are lacking [72, 73]. Subgroup analysis of the FIRST trial in NDMM did not demonstrate a benefit of continuous lenalidomide in HR CA [74]. In relapse MM carfilzomib combined with lenalidomide and dexamethasone combined with carfilzomib (K-RD) were effective across HR and SR patients (23 vs. 29 months, p = NS), while RD showed less activity (13 vs. 19 months, p = 0.004) [75]. Data of IFM did not show a benefit of RD in RRMM with del(13q) or t(4;14) [76]. In the Eloquent-2 trial for RRMM, elotuzumab with RD (E-RD) improved outcome over RD in del(17p) [77]. Recent data of the effect of pomalidomide with dexamethasone in patients with RRMM show that this combination does not abrogate overall adverse outcome in HR-CA, while OS may improve in del(17p) [78]. In Phase 2 trials, a response benefit of pomalidomide with dexamethasone was shown in patients with del(17p) [79]. Hence, lenalidomide seems to partly improve the adverse effect of t(4;14) and del(17p) on PFS but not OS in transplant-eligible patients. In transplant-ineligible patients, there are no data suggesting that the drug may improve outcome with high-risk cytogenetics. Pomalidomide with dexamethasone showed promising results in RRMM with del(17p).

4.5.4   Combined Proteasome Inhibition and Lenalidomide

Bortezomib combined with RD (VRD) in a Phase 1/2 trial in 66 patients with NDMM showed 18-month PFS of 100% in 13 patients with del(17p) and/or t(4;14) [80]. The EVOLUTION trial examined several schedules including VRD in NDMM. One-year PFS was similar in HR-CA (17% of all patients) and SR patients [81]. VRD in transplant-eligible NDMM had similar 3-year PFS (86%) in patients with >60% del(17p) or t(4;14) compared with all patients [82].

Carfilzomib monotherapy did not improve PFS/OS in t(4;14) or del(17p) in RRMM [83]. Carfilzomib combined with pomalidomide/dexamethasone had equivalent PFS and OS in HR vs. SR RRMM [84]. In the Aspire trial in RRMM, KRD was superior to RD for PFS across cytogenetic risk groups, suggesting that this combination (partly) abrogates the negative impact of t(4;14) and del(17p) [75]. Similarly, in TOURMALINE-MM1 ixazomib combined with RD showed identical PFS in patients with del(17p) or t(4;14) or no CA (20 vs. 18 vs. 20 m) [85]. More recently carfilzomib combined with lenalidomide (KRd) or thalidomide (KTd) and dexamethasone in NDMM showed similar CR rate (>60%) and PFS between HR and SR patients [86, 87].

Recently, favorable responses were observed with monoclonal antibodies against CD38 (daratumumab) or SLAMF7 (elotuzumab) combined with Rd in RRMM across cytogenetic subgroups, although data are scarce [88]. In conclusion, combining a proteasome inhibitor with lenalidomide and dexamethasone greatly reduces the adverse effect of t(4;14) and del(17p) on PFS in NDMM. KRd seems effective in patients with high-risk cytogenetics. However, with exception of ASPIRE and TOURMALINE-MM1 most data were obtained in nonrandomized studies, and long-term follow-up has not been reported. NDMM patients with high-risk cytogenetics probably have the highest benefit from the combination of a proteasome inhibitor with lenalidomide or pomalidomide and dexamethasone (Tables 4.3, 4.4, and 4.5).

4.5.5 High-Dose Therapy and ASCT

In transplant-eligible NDMM, the hallmark of first-line treatment is high-dose therapy and ASCT combined with novel agents. This strategy has significantly improved PFS and OS in the past decade. Therefore, it is difficult to address the role of HDT/ASCT for HR-CA. Recently a retrospective analysis in patients without TP53 deletion treated with an autologous transplant did not show a benefit of proteasome inhibitor induction [89]. Few studies have investigated the effect of a second ASCT. In Total Therapy 3 addition of bortezomib to double ASCT improved outcome in patients with t(4;14), indicating that the effect of HDT/ASCT varies with induction and consolidation/maintenance [6]. Similarly, addition of RVD for consolidation and maintenance after ASCT may improve PFS in HR MM [90, 91]. A meta-analysis of four European trials showed that double ASCT combined with bortezomib-based treatment partially abrogates poor PFS in patients carrying both t(4;14) and del(17p) [62]. Taken together HDT/ASCT is standard therapy for eligible patients with NDMM. It contributes to improved outcome across prognostic groups. Double HDT/ASCT combined with bortezomib may improve PFS in patients with t(4;14) or del(17p) and in those with both abnormalities. Although results from stratified randomized trials are not available yet, HDT plus (double) ASCT and proteasome inhibitor-based induction treatment is recommended for patients with high-risk cytogenetics.

4.5.6 Allogeneic Stem Cell Transplantation

Allogeneic SCT has been proposed as a treatment for high-risk younger patients including those with t(4;14) and/or del(17p). Data on CA are scarce and partly

Table 4.3 Survival of newly diagnosed MM patients with high-risk FISH compared with those without high-risk FISH [51]

FISH	Np/Na	End point	Therapy	Present	Absent	Comment	Ref.
Conventional therapy							
t(4;14)	42/290	3-year OS	VBMCP	24%	64%	E9486	[16]
	100/616	3-year OS	VAD + ASCT × 2	55%	80%	IFM-99	[24]
	98/414	3-year OS	VAD + ASCT × ½	40%	72%	IFM-2005	[61]
del17p	37/308	3-year OS	VBMCP	32%	68%	E9486	[16]
	58/474	3-year OS	VAD + ASCT × 2	50%	78%	IFM-99	[24]
	119/393	3-year OS	VAD + ASCT × 1	49%	82%	IFM-2005	[61]
Thalidomide							
t(4;14)	57/181	3-year PFS	TD + ASCT × 2 + TD	20%	48%	GIMEMA	[96]
	26/156	3-year OS	VAD + ASCT × 1 + Thal maintenance	44%	79%	HOVON65/GMMG-HD4	[41]
del17p	21/161	3-year OS	VAD + ASCT × 1 + Thal maintenance	17%	79%	HOVON65/GMMG-HD4	[41]
Lenalidomide							
t(4;14)	28/102	Median OS	RD in RRMM	18 months	23 months	MM-016	[97]
	26/158	Median OS	RD in RRMM	9 months	15 months	IFM	[76]
	152/355	Median PFS	Lenalidomide maintenance	27 months	42 months	IFM-2005	[61]
del17p	12/118	Median OS	RD in RRMM	4 months	23 months	MM-016	[97]
	6.6%	Median PFS	Lenalidomide maintenance	29 months	42 months	IFM-2005	[61]
Bortezomib							
t(4;14)	106/401	4-year OS	VD + ASCT × 1	63%	85%	IFM-2005	[61]
	53/183	3-year PFS	VTD + ASCT × 2 + BzTD	65%	61%	GIMEMA	[96]
	24/148	3-year OS	VAD + ASCT × 1 + Bz	66%	82%	HOVON65/GMMG-HD4	[41]
del17p	54/453	4-year OS	VD + ASCT × 1	50%	79%	IFM-2005	[61]
	16/158	3-year OS	VAD + ASCT × 1 + Bz	69%	82%	HOVON65/GMMG-HD4	[41]

Table 4.4 Survival of high-risk genetic subgroups in randomized controlled clinical trials of newly diagnosed MM: effect of treatment modalities and novel drugs [51]

FISH	N1/N2	End point	Arm 1	Arm 2	Arm 1,%	Arm 2,%	Comment	Ref.
t(4;14)	26/24	3-year OS	PAD/ASCT/Thal*	VAD/ASCT/Bz*	44	66	HOVON65/GMMG-HD4	[17]
	98/106	4-year OS	VAD	VD	32	63*	IFM-2005	[61]
	21/23	2-year OS	Thal*	Placebo*	67	87	TT2	[20]
	21/29	2-year OS	Thalidomide-TT2	Bortezomib TT3	67	97*	TT2 vs. TT3	[63]
Del(17p)	21/16	3-year OS	VAD/ASCT/thalidomide	PAD/ASCT/bortezomib*	17	69*	HOVON65/GMMG-HD4	[17]
	119/54	4-year OS	VAD	VD	36	50	IFM-2005	[61]

*$P < 0.05$

Table 4.5 PFS in high-risk cytogenetics in prospective clinical trials with *novel* agents

Drug	Trial	Schedule	Patients (n)	PFS all (months)	PFS High risk	PFS t(4;14) (n)	PFS del17p (n)
Ixazomib [98]	Tourmaline	Ixa-Len/dex vs. Len/dex	360 362	20.6 14.7	HR 0.54 (n = 75)		
Carfilzomib	Aspire [75]	Car-Len/dex vs. Len/dex	396 396	26.3 17.6	HR 0.70 (n = 100)		
	Endeavour [99]	Car/Dex Bor/Dex	464 465	18.7 9.4	HR 0.65 (n = 127)		
Elotuzumab	Eloquent-2 [77]	Elo-Len/dex vs. Len/dex	321 325	19.4 14.9		HR 0.53 (n = 46)	HR 0.65 (n = 111)
Pomalidomide [100]	MM003	Pom/Dex Dex	302 153	4.0 1.9	HR 0.46		
Panobinostat [101]	Panorama 2	Pan-Bor/Dex Bor/Dex	387 381	12 8.1	HR 0.47 (n = 37)		

based on classic karyotyping. In a trial of 73 NDMM patients, tandem auto-allo-transplantation yielded similar 5-year PFS (24% vs. 30%) and OS (50% vs. 54%) in patients without t(4;14) or del(17p) [92]. The EBMT-NMAM2000 study showed better OS in patients treated with ASCT/RIC-allo or ASCT alone, 49% vs. 36% at 96 months, respectively ($P = 0.030$). Unfortunately, convincing FISH data are lacking [93]. A retrospective analysis in 143 patients indicated that patients with del(13q) or t(4;14) or del(17p) or t(11;14) had similar 3-year PFS and OS as patients without any abnormality [94]. A study of allo-SCT in 101 relapsed MM showed worse 4-year PFS (28 vs. 43%) and OS (30 vs. 49%) in 16 patients with del(17p), while in 16 patients with t(4;14), no impact was observed [95]. At this stage it should be concluded that data are limited and that allogeneic SCT or tandem auto-allo-SCT may possibly improve PFS in patients with t(4;14) or del(17p). Results are better in an early stage of the disease. The novel treatments may challenge the role of allo-SCT, and this treatment modality should currently only be used to clinical trials.

Conclusions

Risk stratification in MM is important to predict survival and to define a treatment strategy. Cytogenetic abnormalities by FISH currently are clinically relevant prognostic factors in MM. The IMWG consensus panel on FISH advises to test for the presence of del(17p), t(4;14), and possibly t(14;16). An extended panel, which may be incorporated in clinical trials, includes t(11;14), t(14;20), gain(1q), del(1p), del(13q), and ploidy status. Bortezomib and lenalidomide may partially abrogate the adverse effect of del(17p). Bortezomib combined with iMIDS may improve outcome in t(4;14). Double HDT/ASCT plus bortezomib may improve outcome in patients with both adverse CA. Application of these risk factors may be a first step toward precision medicine in patients with MM.

Disclosures PS   Research support: Amgen/Onyx, Celgene, Janssen, Karyopharm, SkylineDx
Honoraria: Amgen/Onyx, Celgene, Janssen, Karyopharm

References

1. Palumbo A, Anderson K. Multiple myeloma. N Engl J Med. 2011;364(11):1046–60.
2. Rajkumar SV, Dimopoulos MA, Palumbo A, et al. International Myeloma Working Group updated criteria for the diagnosis of multiple myeloma. Lancet Oncol. 2014;15(12):E538–48.
3. Morgan GJ, Walker BA, Davies FE. The genetic architecture of multiple myeloma. Nat Rev Cancer. 2012;12(5):335–48.
4. Avet-Loiseau H, Magrangeas F, Moreau P, et al. Molecular heterogeneity of multiple myeloma: pathogenesis, prognosis, and therapeutic implications. J Clin Oncol. 2011;29(14):1893–7.
5. Sonneveld P, Avet-Loiseau H, Lonial S, et al. Treatment of multiple myeloma with high-risk cytogenetics: a consensus of the International Myeloma Working Group. Blood. 2016;127(24):2955–62.
6. Usmani SZ, Crowley J, Hoering A, et al. Improvement in long-term outcomes with successive Total Therapy trials for multiple myeloma: are patients now being cured? Leukemia. 2013;27(1):226–32.

7. Ross FM, Avet-Loiseau H, Ameye G, et al. Report from the European Myeloma Network on interphase FISH in multiple myeloma and related disorders. Haematologica. 2012;97(8):1272–7.

8. Avet-Loiseau H, Munshi N, Li C, et al. Use of high-density SNP-array analysis to identify novel chromosomal abnormalities that predict survival in multiple myeloma. J Clin Oncol 2008;26(15).

9. Gertz MA, Lacy MQ, Dispenzieri A, et al. Clinical implications of t(11;14)(q13;q32), t(4;14)(p16.3;q32), and -17p13 in myeloma patients treated with high-dose therapy. Blood. 2005;106(8):2837–40.

10. Bergsagel PL, Kuehl WM, Zhan F, Sawyer J, Barlogie B, Shaughnessy J Jr. Cyclin D dysregulation: an early and unifying pathogenic event in multiple myeloma. Blood. 2005;106(1):296–303.

11. Chng WJ, Chung TH, Kumar S, et al. Gene signature combinations improve prognostic stratification of multiple myeloma patients. Leukemia. 2015;30(5):1071–8.

12. Munshi NC, Avet-Loiseau H. Genomics in multiple myeloma. Clin Cancer Res. 2011;17(6):1234–42.

13. Kuehl WM, Bergsagel PL. Multiple myeloma: evolving genetic events and host interactions. Nat Rev Cancer. 2002;2(3):175–87.

14. Neben K, Jauch A, Bertsch U, et al. Combining information regarding chromosomal aberrations t(4;14) and del(17p13) with the International Staging System classification allows stratification of myeloma patients undergoing autologous stem cell transplantation. Haematologica. 2010;95(7):1150–7.

15. Boyd KD, Ross FM, Chiecchio L, et al. A novel prognostic model in myeloma based on co-segregating adverse FISH lesions and the ISS: analysis of patients treated in the MRC Myeloma IX trial. Leukemia. 2012;26(2):349–55.

16. Fonseca R, Blood E, Rue M, et al. Clinical and biologic implications of recurrent genomic aberrations in myeloma. Blood. 2003;101(11):4569–75.

17. Sonneveld P, Schmidt-Wolf IG, van der Holt B, et al. Bortezomib induction and maintenance treatment in patients with newly diagnosed multiple myeloma: results of the randomized phase III HOVON-65/GMMG-HD4 trial. J Clin Oncol. 2012;30(24):2946–55.

18. Sonneveld P, Goldschmidt H, Rosinol L, et al. Bortezomib-based versus nonbortezomib-based induction treatment before autologous stem-cell transplantation in patients with previously untreated multiple myeloma: a meta-analysis of phase III randomized, controlled trials. J Clin Oncol. 2013;31(26):3279–87.

19. Cavo M, Tacchetti P, Patriarca F, et al. Bortezomib with thalidomide plus dexamethasone compared with thalidomide plus dexamethasone as induction therapy before, and consolidation therapy after, double autologous stem-cell transplantation in newly diagnosed multiple myeloma: a randomised phase 3 study. Lancet. 2010;376(9758):2075–85.

20. Barlogie B, Pineda-Roman M, van Rhee F, et al. Thalidomide arm of Total Therapy 2 improves complete remission duration and survival in myeloma patients with metaphase cytogenetic abnormalities. Blood. 2008;112(8):3115–21.

21. Moreau P, Attal M, Garban F, et al. Heterogeneity of t(4;14) in multiple myeloma. Long-term follow-up of 100 cases treated with tandem transplantation in IFM99 trials. Leukemia. 2007;21(9):2020–4.

22. Shaughnessy JD Jr, Zhan F, Burington BE, et al. A validated gene expression model of high-risk multiple myeloma is defined by deregulated expression of genes mapping to chromosome 1. Blood. 2007;109(6):2276–84.

23. Hebraud B, Magrangeas F, Cleynen A, et al. Role of additional chromosomal changes in the prognostic value of t(4;14) and del(17p) in multiple myeloma: the IFM experience. Blood. 2015;125(13):2095–100.

24. Avet-Loiseau H, Attal M, Moreau P, et al. Genetic abnormalities and survival in multiple myeloma: the experience of the Intergroupe Francophone du Myelome. Blood. 2007;109(8):3489–95.

25. Pawlyn C, Melchor L, Murison A, et al. Coexistent hyperdiploidy does not abrogate poor prognosis in myeloma with adverse cytogenetics and may precede IGH translocations. Blood. 2015;125(5):831–40.
26. Walker BA, Leone PE, Chiecchio L, et al. A compendium of myeloma-associated chromosomal copy number abnormalities and their prognostic value. Blood. 2010;116(15):e56–65.
27. Fonseca R, Bergsagel PL, Drach J, et al. International Myeloma Working Group molecular classification of multiple myeloma: spotlight review. Leukemia. 2009;23(12):2210–21.
28. Teoh PJ, Chung TH, Sebastian S, et al. p53 haploinsufficiency and functional abnormalities in multiple myeloma. Leukemia. 2014;28(10):2066–74.
29. Walker BA, Boyle EM, Wardell CP, et al. Mutational spectrum, copy number changes, and outcome: results of a sequencing study of patients with newly diagnosed myeloma. J Clin Oncol. 2015;33(33):3911–20.
30. Billecke L, Murga Penas EM, May AM, et al. Cytogenetics of extramedullary manifestations in multiple myeloma. Br J Haematol. 2013;161(1):87–94.
31. Lopez-Anglada L, Gutierrez NC, Garcia JL, Mateos MV, Flores T, San Miguel JF. P53 deletion may drive the clinical evolution and treatment response in multiple myeloma. Eur J Haematol. 2010;84(4):359–61.
32. Morgan GJ, Gregory WM, Davies FE, et al. The role of maintenance thalidomide therapy in multiple myeloma: MRC Myeloma IX results and meta-analysis. Blood. 2012;119(1):7–15.
33. Kumar S, Fonseca R, Ketterling RP, et al. Trisomies in multiple myeloma: impact on survival in patients with high-risk cytogenetics. Blood. 2012;119(9):2100–5.
34. Ludwig H, Durie BG, Bolejack V, et al. Myeloma in patients younger than age 50 years presents with more favorable features and shows better survival: an analysis of 10,549 patients from the International Myeloma Working Group. Blood. 2008;111(8):4039–47.
35. Gay F, Larocca A, Wijermans P, et al. Complete response correlates with long-term progression-free and overall survival in elderly myeloma treated with novel agents: analysis of 1175 patients. Blood. 2011;117(11):3025–31.
36. Stewart AK, Bergsagel PL, Greipp PR, et al. A practical guide to defining high-risk myeloma for clinical trials, patient counseling and choice of therapy. Leukemia. 2007;21(3):529–34.
37. Rajkumar SV, Gahrton G, Bergsagel PL. Approach to the treatment of multiple myeloma: a clash of philosophies. Blood. 2011;118(12):3205–11.
38. Gutierrez NC, Castellanos MV, Martin ML, et al. Prognostic and biological implications of genetic abnormalities in multiple myeloma undergoing autologous stem cell transplantation: t(4;14) is the most relevant adverse prognostic factor, whereas RB deletion as a unique abnormality is not associated with adverse prognosis. Leukemia. 2007;21(1):143–50.
39. Chng WJ, Dispenzieri A, Chim CS, et al. IMWG consensus on risk stratification in multiple myeloma. Leukemia. 2014;28(2):269–77.
40. Avet-Loiseau H, Durie BG, Cavo M, et al. Combining fluorescent in situ hybridization data with ISS staging improves risk assessment in myeloma: an International Myeloma Working Group collaborative project. Leukemia. 2013;27(3):711–7.
41. Neben K, Lokhorst HM, Jauch A, et al. Administration of bortezomib before and after autologous stem cell transplantation improves outcome in multiple myeloma patients with deletion 17p. Blood. 2012;119(4):940–8.
42. Moreau P, Cavo M, Sonneveld P, et al. Combination of international scoring system 3, high lactate dehydrogenase, and t(4;14) and/or del(17p) identifies patients with multiple myeloma (MM) treated with front-line autologous stem-cell transplantation at high risk of early MM progression-related death. J Clin Oncol. 2014;32(20):2173–80.
43. Palumbo A, Avet-Loiseau H, Oliva S, et al. Revised International Staging System for Multiple Myeloma: a report from International Myeloma Working Group. J Clin Oncol. 2015;33(26):2863–9.
44. Zhan F, Hardin J, Kordsmeier B, et al. Global gene expression profiling of multiple myeloma, monoclonal gammopathy of undetermined significance, and normal bone marrow plasma cells. Blood. 2002;99(5):1745–57.

45. Shaughnessy JD Jr, Qu P, Usmani S, et al. Pharmacogenomics of bortezomib test-dosing identifies hyperexpression of proteasome genes, especially PSMD4, as novel high-risk feature in myeloma treated with Total Therapy 3. Blood. 2011;118(13):3512–24.
46. Kuiper R, Broyl A, de Knegt Y, et al. A gene expression signature for high-risk multiple myeloma. Leukemia. 2012;26(11):2406–13.
47. Kuiper R, van Duin M, van Vliet MH, et al. Prediction of high- and low-risk multiple myeloma based on gene expression and the International Staging System. Blood. 2015.
48. Decaux O, Lode L, Magrangeas F, et al. Prediction of survival in multiple myeloma based on gene expression profiles reveals cell cycle and chromosomal instability signatures in high-risk patients and hyperdiploid signatures in low-risk patients: a study of the Intergroupe Francophone du Myelome. J Clin Oncol. 2008;26(29):4798–805.
49. Amin SB, Yip WK, Minvielle S, et al. Gene expression profile alone is inadequate in predicting complete response in multiple myeloma. Leukemia. 2014;28(11):2229–34.
50. Mikhael JR, Dingli D, Roy V, et al. Management of newly diagnosed symptomatic multiple myeloma: updated Mayo Stratification of Myeloma and Risk-Adapted Therapy (mSMART) consensus guidelines 2013. Mayo Clin Proc. 2013;88(4):360–76.
51. Bergsagel PL, Mateos MV, Gutierrez NC, Rajkumar SV, San Miguel JF. Improving overall survival and overcoming adverse prognosis in the treatment of cytogenetically high-risk multiple myeloma. Blood. 2013;121(6):884–92.
52. Bianchi G, Richardson PG, Anderson KC. Best treatment strategies in high-risk multiple myeloma: navigating a gray area. J Clin Oncol. 2014;32(20):2125–32.
53. Singhal S, Mehta J, Desikan R, et al. Antitumor activity of thalidomide in refractory multiple myeloma. N Engl J Med. 1999;341(21):1565–71.
54. Morgan GJ, Davies FE, Gregory WM, et al. Cyclophosphamide, thalidomide, and dexamethasone (CTD) as initial therapy for patients with multiple myeloma unsuitable for autologous transplantation. Blood. 2011;118(5):1231–8.
55. Morgan GJ, Davies FE, Gregory WM, et al. Cyclophosphamide, thalidomide, and dexamethasone as induction therapy for newly diagnosed multiple myeloma patients destined for autologous stem-cell transplantation: MRC Myeloma IX randomized trial results. Haematologica. 2012;97(3):442–50.
56. Rosinol L, Oriol A, Teruel AI, et al. Superiority of bortezomib, thalidomide, and dexamethasone (VTD) as induction pretransplantation therapy in multiple myeloma: a randomized phase 3 PETHEMA/GEM study. Blood. 2012;120(8):1589–96.
57. Lokhorst HM, van der Holt B, Zweegman S, et al. A randomized phase 3 study on the effect of thalidomide combined with adriamycin, dexamethasone, and high-dose melphalan, followed by thalidomide maintenance in patients with multiple myeloma. Blood. 2010;115(6):1113–20.
58. Attal M, Harousseau JL, Leyvraz S, et al. Maintenance therapy with thalidomide improves survival in patients with multiple myeloma. Blood. 2006;108(10):3289–94.
59. Boyd KD, Ross FM, Tapper WJ, et al. The clinical impact and molecular biology of del(17p) in multiple myeloma treated with conventional or thalidomide-based therapy. Genes Chromosomes Cancer. 2011;50(10):765–74.
60. Barlogie B, Anaissie E, van Rhee F, et al. The Arkansas approach to therapy of patients with multiple myeloma. Best Pract Res Clin Haematol. 2007;20(4):761–81.
61. Avet-Loiseau H, Leleu X, Roussel M, et al. Bortezomib plus dexamethasone induction improves outcome of patients with t(4;14) myeloma but not outcome of patients with del(17p). J Clin Oncol. 2010;28(30):4630–4.
62. Cavo M, Salwender H, Rosinol L, et al. Double vs single autologous stem cell transplantation after bortezomib-based induction regimens for multiple myeloma: an integrated analysis of patient-level data from phase European III studies. Blood 2013;122(21).
63. Nair B, van Rhee F, Shaughnessy JD Jr, et al. Superior results of Total Therapy 3 (2003-33) in gene expression profiling-defined low-risk multiple myeloma confirmed in subsequent trial 2006-66 with VRD maintenance. Blood. 2010;115(21):4168–73.

64. Pineda-Roman M, Zangari M, Haessler J, et al. Sustained complete remissions in multiple myeloma linked to bortezomib in total therapy 3: comparison with total therapy 2. Br J Haematol. 2008;140(6):625–34.
65. San Miguel JF, Schlag R, Khuageva NK, et al. Bortezomib plus melphalan and prednisone for initial treatment of multiple myeloma. N Engl J Med. 2008;359(9):906–17.
66. Mateos MV, Gutierrez NC, Martin-Ramos ML, et al. Outcome according to cytogenetic abnormalities and DNA ploidy in myeloma patients receiving short induction with weekly bortezomib followed by maintenance. Blood. 2011;118(17):4547–53.
67. Palumbo APBS, Rossi D, Berretta S, Montefusco V, Peccatori J, et al. A phase III study of VMPT versus VMP in newly diagnosed elderly myeloma patients. J Clin Oncol. 2009;27:8515a.
68. Avet-Loiseau H, Hulin C, Campion L, et al. Chromosomal abnormalities are major prognostic factors in elderly patients with multiple myeloma: the intergroupe francophone du myelome experience. J Clin Oncol. 2013;31(22):2806–9.
69. Kapoor P, Kumar S, Fonseca R, et al. Impact of risk stratification on outcome among patients with multiple myeloma receiving initial therapy with lenalidomide and dexamethasone. Blood. 2009;114(3):518–21.
70. Palumbo A, Cavallo F, Gay F, et al. Autologous transplantation and maintenance therapy in multiple myeloma. N Engl J Med. 2014;371(10):895–905.
71. Attal M, Lauwers-Cances V, Marit G, et al. Lenalidomide maintenance after stem-cell transplantation for multiple myeloma. N Engl J Med. 2012;366(19):1782–91.
72. Palumbo A, Hajek R, Delforge M, et al. Continuous lenalidomide treatment for newly diagnosed multiple myeloma. N Engl J Med. 2012;366(19):1759–69.
73. McCarthy PL, Owzar K, Hofmeister CC, et al. Lenalidomide after stem-cell transplantation for multiple myeloma. N Engl J Med. 2012;366(19):1770–81.
74. Benboubker L, Dimopoulos MA, Dispenzieri A, et al. Lenalidomide and dexamethasone in transplant-ineligible patients with myeloma. N Engl J Med. 2014;371(10):906–17.
75. Stewart AK, Rajkumar SV, Dimopoulos MA, et al. Carfilzomib, lenalidomide, and dexamethasone for relapsed multiple myeloma. N Engl J Med. 2015;372(2):142–52.
76. Avet-Loiseau H, Soulier J, Fermand JP, et al. Impact of high-risk cytogenetics and prior therapy on outcomes in patients with advanced relapsed or refractory multiple myeloma treated with lenalidomide plus dexamethasone. Leukemia. 2010;24(3):623–8.
77. Lonial S, Dimopoulos M, Palumbo A, et al. Elotuzumab therapy for relapsed or refractory multiple myeloma. N Engl J Med. 2015;373(7):621–31.
78. Dimopoulos MA, Weisel KC, Song KW, et al. Cytogenetics and long-term survival of patients with refractory or relapsed and refractory multiple myeloma treated with pomalidomide and low-dose dexamethasone. Haematologica. 2015;100(10):1327–33.
79. Leleu X, Karlin L, Macro M, et al. Pomalidomide plus low-dose dexamethasone in multiple myeloma with deletion 17p and/or translocation (4;14): IFM 2010-02 trial results. Blood. 2015;125(9):1411–7.
80. Richardson PG, Weller E, Lonial S, et al. Lenalidomide, bortezomib, and dexamethasone combination therapy in patients with newly diagnosed multiple myeloma. Blood. 2010;116(5):679–86.
81. Kumar S, Flinn I, Richardson PG, et al. Randomized, multicenter, phase 2 study (EVOLUTION) of combinations of bortezomib, dexamethasone, cyclophosphamide, and lenalidomide in previously untreated multiple myeloma. Blood. 2012;119(19):4375–82.
82. Roussel M, Lauwers-Cances V, Robillard N, et al. Front-line transplantation program with lenalidomide, bortezomib, and dexamethasone combination as induction and consolidation followed by lenalidomide maintenance in patients with multiple myeloma: a phase II study by the Intergroupe Francophone du Myelome. J Clin Oncol. 2014;32(25):2712–7.
83. Jakubowiak AJ, Siegel DS, Martin T, et al. Treatment outcomes in patients with relapsed and refractory multiple myeloma and high-risk cytogenetics receiving single-agent carfilzomib in the PX-171-003-A1 study. Leukemia. 2013;27(12):2351–6.

84. Shah JJ, Stadtmauer EA, Abonour R, et al. Carfilzomib, pomalidomide, and dexamethasone (CPD) in patients with relapsed and/or refractory multiple myeloma. Blood. 2015.
85. Moreau P Masszi T GNea. Ixazomib, an Investigational Oral Proteasome Inhibitor (PI), in Combination with Lenalidomide and Dexamethasone (IRd), Significantly Extends Progression-Free Survival (PFS) for Patients (Pts) with Relapsed and/or Refractory Multiple Myeloma (RRMM): the phase 3 tourmaline-MM1 study (NCT01564537) Abstract 727. Blood. 2015;126(23).
86. Sonneveld P, Asselbergs E, Zweegman S, et al. Phase 2 study of carfilzomib, thalidomide, and dexamethasone as induction/consolidation therapy for newly diagnosed multiple myeloma. Blood. 2015;125(3):449–56.
87. Jakubowiak AJ, Dytfeld D, Griffith KA, et al. A phase 1/2 study of carfilzomib in combination with lenalidomide and low-dose dexamethasone as a frontline treatment for multiple myeloma. Blood. 2012;120(9):1801–9.
88. van de Donk NW, Moreau P, Plesner T, et al. Clinical efficacy and management of monoclonal antibodies targeting CD38 and SLAMF7 in multiple myeloma. Blood. 2015;127(6):681–95.
89. Gaballa S, Saliba RM, Srour S, et al. Outcomes in patients with multiple myeloma with TP53 deletion after autologous hematopoietic stem cell transplant. Am J Hematol. 2016.
90. Nooka AK, Kastritis E, Dimopoulos MA, Lonial S. Treatment options for relapsed and refractory multiple myeloma. Blood. 2015;125(20):3085–99.
91. Nooka AK, Kaufman JL, Muppidi S, et al. Consolidation and maintenance therapy with lenalidomide, bortezomib and dexamethasone (RVD) in high-risk myeloma patients. Leukemia. 2014;28(3):690–3.
92. Kroger N, Badbaran A, Zabelina T, et al. Impact of high-risk cytogenetics and achievement of molecular remission on long-term freedom from disease after autologous-allogeneic tandem transplantation in patients with multiple myeloma. Biol Blood Marrow Transplant. 2013;19(3):398–404.
93. Gahrton G, Iacobelli S, Bjorkstrand B, et al. Autologous/reduced-intensity allogeneic stem cell transplantation vs autologous transplantation in multiple myeloma: long-term results of the EBMT-NMAM2000 study. Blood. 2013;121(25):5055–63.
94. Roos-Weil D, Moreau P, Avet-Loiseau H, et al. Impact of genetic abnormalities after allogeneic stem cell transplantation in multiple myeloma: a report of the Societe Francaise de Greffe de Moelle et de Therapie Cellulaire. Haematologica. 2011;96(10):1504–11.
95. Schilling G, Hansen T, Shimoni A, et al. Impact of genetic abnormalities on survival after allogeneic hematopoietic stem cell transplantation in multiple myeloma. Leukemia. 2008;22(6):1250–5.
96. Cavo M, Pantani L, Petrucci MT, et al. Bortezomib-thalidomide-dexamethasone is superior to thalidomide-dexamethasone as consolidation therapy after autologous hematopoietic stem cell transplantation in patients with newly diagnosed multiple myeloma. Blood. 2012;120(1):9–19.
97. Reece D, Song KW, Fu T, et al. Influence of cytogenetics in patients with relapsed or refractory multiple myeloma treated with lenalidomide plus dexamethasone: adverse effect of deletion 17p13. Blood. 2009;114(3):522–5.
98. Moreau P, Masszi T, Grzasko N, et al. Oral ixazomib, lenalidomide, and dexamethasone for multiple myeloma. N Engl J Med. 2016;374(17):1621–34.
99. Dimopoulos MA, Moreau P, Palumbo A, Chng WJ, Feng S. Carfilozomib versus bortezomib for relapsed or refractory myeloma—authors' reply. Lancet Oncol. 2016;17(4):e126.
100. San Miguel J, Weisel K, Moreau P, et al. Pomalidomide plus low-dose dexamethasone versus high-dose dexamethasone alone for patients with relapsed and refractory multiple myeloma (MM-003): a randomised, open-label, phase 3 trial. Lancet Oncol. 2013;14(11):1055–66.
101. San-Miguel JF, Hungria VT, Yoon SS, et al. Panobinostat plus bortezomib and dexamethasone versus placebo plus bortezomib and dexamethasone in patients with relapsed or relapsed and refractory multiple myeloma: a multicentre, randomised, double-blind phase 3 trial. Lancet Oncol. 2014;15(11):1195–206.

Treatment of Patients in First or Second Relapse

5

Andrew J. Yee and Noopur S. Raje

5.1 Introduction

While multiple myeloma remains incurable, the past decade has seen dramatic advances with the introduction of immunomodulatory drugs (IMiDs) and proteasome inhibitors (PI). The adoption of these newer drugs has significantly improved overall survival. Patients who relapsed after 2000 had a doubling of overall survival from 11.8 months for disease relapse prior to 2000 to 23.9 months [1]. Recently, next-generation IMiDs (pomalidomide) and PIs (carfilzomib, ixazomib) have been approved along with drugs with new mechanisms of action, such as the HDAC inhibitor panobinostat and the monoclonal antibodies elotuzumab and daratumumab. This chapter will focus on the approach to patients who develop a relapse after one or two lines of treatment.

5.2 Definitions of Relapse

The International Myeloma Working Group (IMWG) has defined criteria for disease progression and several categories of relapsed disease. It has defined "relapsed disease" as previously treated myeloma that progresses and requires initiation of treatment but does not meet criteria for "primary refractory myeloma" or "relapsed and refractory myeloma" [2]. There are several criteria for disease progression, based on an increase of 25% from the lowest response value in any of the following:

A.J. Yee • N.S. Raje (✉)
Center for Multiple Myeloma, Massachusetts General Hospital Cancer Center, Boston, MA 02114, USA

Harvard Medical School, Boston, MA 02115, USA
e-mail: ayee1@mgh.harvard.edu; nraje@mgh.harvard.edu

© Springer International Publishing AG 2018
S.Z. Usmani, A.K. Nooka (eds.), *Personalized Therapy for Multiple Myeloma*,
https://doi.org/10.1007/978-3-319-61872-2_5

1. Serum M-component (absolute increase must be ≥0.5 g/dL)
2. Urine M-component (absolute increase must be ≥200 mg/24 h)
3. In patients without measurable serum or urine M protein levels:
   (a) Difference between involved and involved free light chain values (absolute increase must be >10 mg/dL)
      • In patients without measurable serum, urine M protein, or free light chain values, bone marrow plasma cell percentage (absolute percentage must be ≥10%)
4. Definite development of new bone lesions or soft tissue plasmacytomas or definite increase in size of existing bone lesions or soft tissue plasmacytomas
5. Development of hypercalcemia (corrected serum calcium >11.5 mg/dL) that can be attributed solely to the plasma cell proliferative disorder

"Relapsed and refractory myeloma" is defined as a disease that is nonresponsive while on salvage therapy or progressed within 60 days of last therapy in patients who have achieved minimal response or better at some point previously. "Primary refractory" disease is defined as a disease that is nonresponsive in patients who have never achieved a minimal response or better with any therapy.

There are also proposed guidelines for defining the number of lines of therapy as well [3]. For example, a planned sequential course of therapy with induction chemotherapy, followed by stem cell transplant, and lenalidomide maintenance is considered one line of treatment.

Clinical relapse. The IMWG has defined "clinical relapse" as symptomatic disease related to disease progression on two consecutive assessments [4]:

1. Development of new soft tissue plasmacytomas or bone lesions on imaging
2. Increase in the size of existing plasmacytomas or bone lesions of 50% (and >1 cm)
3. Hypercalcemia (>11.5 mg/dL)
4. Decrease in hemoglobin of >2 g/dL or hemoglobin <10 g/dL
5. Rise in serum creatinine by ≥2 mg/dL
6. Hyperviscosity

Significant paraprotein relapse. The IMWG defined significant paraprotein relapse to identify patients where the rate or magnitude of change in monoclonal protein or free light chain may, in the absence of symptoms, warrant initiation of treatment:

1. Doubling of the M-component in two consecutive measurements separated ≤2 months
2. Increase in the absolute level of serum M protein by ≥1 g/dL
3. Increase in urine M protein by ≥500 mg/24 h
4. Increase in involved free light chain level by ≥20 mg/dL (plus an abnormal FLC ratio) in two consecutive measurements separated by ≤2 months

5.3   Timing of Treatment

While patients who have symptoms related to their disease progression, i.e., clinical relapse, generally require treatment at that time, in patients with an asymptomatic rise in monoclonal protein, the IMWG provides guidelines for the timing of initiating treatment based on the above criteria for significant paraprotein relapse. Of note, a series examining patterns of relapse in 211 patients after autologous stem cell transplant noted that there was a wide range between onset of asymptomatic relapse (or biochemical relapse) and progression and treatment, varying from 0 to 5.6 years, with a median of 5.6 months [5]. The clinical features of relapse were generally similar to the features at time of presentation, e.g., patients who relapsed with renal impairment tended to have renal impairment at time of diagnosis. Notably, 26% of patients with asymptomatic relapse did not require treatment for at least 2 years, suggesting that there is a group of patients with biochemical relapse who may follow a more indolent course.

5.4   Immunomodulatory Drugs

5.4.1 Lenalidomide

Lenalidomide is a second-generation IMiD with a chemical structure similar to thalidomide, and it is widely used at all stages of illness. The specific mechanism of action of IMiDs has only recently been determined. IMiDs as a class bind to cereblon, a component of E3 ubiquitin ligase complexes. This complex then promotes the degradation of transcription factors critical to MM proliferation: IKZF1/3, MYC, and IRF4 [6–8]. Compared to thalidomide, lenalidomide is associated with significantly less peripheral neuropathy, sedation, and constipation but is associated with more myelosuppression. Two phase III trials, MM-009 [9] and MM-010 [10] (Table 5.1), showed that the combination of lenalidomide and dexamethasone was superior to dexamethasone alone and established the role for lenalidomide in relapsed disease. These trials shared a similar design: lenalidomide was given as 25 mg daily on days 1–21 on a 28-day cycle with dexamethasone 40 mg on days 1–4, 9–12, and 17–20 for the first four cycles and then on days 1–4. About two-thirds of patients had two or more prior lines of therapy. Pooling these trials together, the combination had a higher overall response rate (i.e., partial response or better; ORR), 60.6% vs. 21.9% [20]. The median time to progression and overall survival were also higher, 13.4 vs. 4.6 months and at least 38 months vs. 31.6 months, respectively. The benefit in survival was seen even when 47.6% of patients randomized to the dexamethasone alone arm crossed over after disease progression or study unblinding. Given these findings, lenalidomide was approved by the FDA for treating relapsed disease in June 2006.

Notable side effects seen in the lenalidomide arm included grade 3–4 neutropenia, roughly 29.5–41.2%, and grade 3–4 venous thromboembolic (VTE) events, 11.4–14.7%. Of note, in these trials, prophylaxis with aspirin was not mandated, as

Table 5.1 Selected phase III trials in relapsed disease

Reference	Name of trial	Arm	N	PFS[a]	HR	ORR (%)	≥VGPR (%)	≥CR (%)
Palumbo et al. [11]	CASTOR	Dara-Vd	251	NE	0.39	83	59	19
		Vd	247	7.2		63	29	9
Dimopoulos et al. [12]	POLLUX	Dara-Rd	286	NE	0.37	93	76	43
		Rd	283	18.4		76	44	19
Dimopoulos et al. [13]	ENDEAVOR	Kd	464	18.7	0.53	77	54	13
		Vd	465	9.4		63	29	6
Moreau et al. [14]	TOURMALINE-MM1	IRd	360	20.6	0.74	78	48	12
		Rd	362	14.7		72	39	7
Lonial et al. [15]	ELOQUENT-2	Elo-Rd	321	19.4	0.7	79	33	4
		Rd	325	14.9		66	28	7
Stewart et al. [16]	ASPIRE	KRd	396	26.3	0.69	87	70	32
		Rd	396	17.6		67	40	9
San-Miguel et al. [17]	PANORAMA 1	Pano-Vd	387	12.71	0.63	61		11
		Vd	381	8.54		55		6
San Miguel et al. [18]	NIMBUS (MM-003)	Pd	302	3.8	0.41	31	6	1
		D	153	1.9		10	1	0
Weber et al. [9]	MM-009	RD	177	11.4[b]		61		14
		D	176	4.7		20		1
Dimopoulos et al. [10]	MM-010	RD	176	11.3[b]		60		16
		D	175	4.7		24		3
Richardson et al. [19]	APEX	V	333	6.22[b]		38		6
		D	336	3.49		18		1

D high-dose dexamethasone, *d* low-dose dexamethasone, *dara* daratumumab, *elo* elotuzumab, *I* ixazomib, *K* carfilzomib, *P* pomalidomide, *Pano* panobinostat, *R* lenalidomide, *V* bortezomib
[a]PFS is in months
[b]Time to progression

is currently the recommended practice [21, 22]. Furthermore, current practice has moved to using lower doses of dexamethasone (40 mg weekly), based on the results of the ECOG E403 study [23], which showed that the rate of VTE was significantly lower with the low-dose dexamethasone regimen (12%) compared to the traditional high-dose regimen (26%) ($p = 0.0003$). Of note, in this study, VTE prophylaxis was recommended but not mandated initially in the study. Additionally, development of a second primary malignancy is an increasingly appreciated risk of lenalidomide therapy. A meta-analysis of nine randomized trials in newly diagnosed patients found that the cumulative incidence of all second primary malignancies was 6.9% in the lenalidomide arm vs. 4.8% in the control arm ($p = 0.037$) [24]. However, the risk of a second malignancy may be less relevant in the relapsed setting.

Given the increasing use of lenalidomide in the up-front setting (as a doublet with dexamethasone or in combination with, e.g., bortezomib) as well as increasing adoption of lenalidomide maintenance after induction chemotherapy or autologous stem cell transplant, the role for a traditional lenalidomide-dexamethasone doublet for relapsed disease may be less than in the past. Rather, other regimens (or a triplet combination with lenalidomide) may be more attractive, as detailed below.

5.4.2 Pomalidomide

Pomalidomide is a third-generation IMiD, and it is effective in patients with disease refractory to lenalidomide. The MM-002 study was a phase II study where patients with relapsed and refractory MM and who had two or more prior lines were randomized to receive pomalidomide alone (4 mg on days 1–21 of a 28-day cycle) or pomalidomide with low-dose dexamethasone (40 mg weekly) [25]. All patients had received prior treatment with at least two cycles of lenalidomide and at least two cycles of bortezomib. The ORR was 33% in the pomalidomide-dexamethasone arm compared to 18% in the pomalidomide alone arm ($p = 0.013$). Progression-free survival (PFS) and overall survival (OS) were also higher in the doublet arm, 4.2 vs. 2.7 months ($p = 0.003$) and 16.5 vs. 13.6 months, respectively. Importantly, refractoriness to lenalidomide or both lenalidomide and bortezomib did not affect the response to pomalidomide.

These findings were further extended in the MM-003 study, a phase III study comparing pomalidomide and dexamethasone to high-dose dexamethasone [18]. This study enrolled patients with refractory disease who received at least two previous consecutive cycles of bortezomib and lenalidomide, alone or in combination and who had adequate alkylator treatment (e.g., as part of an autologous stem cell transplant). Patients in the trial had received a median of five prior lines of treatment. The ORR was significantly higher in the pomalidomide-dexamethasone arm, 31% vs. 10% in the high-dose dexamethasone arm ($p < 0.0001$). The median PFS with pomalidomide plus low-dose dexamethasone was 3.8 vs. 1.9 months ($p < 0.0001$). Adjusting for crossover, the median OS was 12.7 vs. 5.7 months [26]. While high-dose dexamethasone alone is not conventionally used in the USA, the MM-003 study demonstrated effectiveness of pomalidomide and low-dose dexamethasone in patients refractory to lenalidomide and bortezomib. Based on the findings in MM-002 and MM-003, pomalidomide with low-dose dexamethasone was approved by the FDA in February 2013 for patients with refractory disease and who have received at least two prior therapies including lenalidomide and a PI.

Similar to lenalidomide, myelosuppression is a common characteristic of pomalidomide, with 41% and 48% of patients experiencing grade 3–4 neutropenia in the MM-002 and MM-003 trials, respectively. In the MM-002 trial, 46% of patients in the pomalidomide and low-dose dexamethasone arm received G-CSF. On the other hand, there are several notable differences with pomalidomide compared with lenalidomide. Unlike lenalidomide, pomalidomide is extensively metabolized prior to excretion, and thus dosing of pomalidomide is not as dependent on renal function as lenalidomide [27], though patients with creatinine >3 mg/dL were excluded in clinical studies. In the MM-010 study, a phase IIIb study of pomalidomide and low-dose dexamethasone with a similar patient population as MM-003, the safety and efficacy of this regimen were similar in patients with moderate renal impairment (creatinine clearance 45–60 mL/min) compared to patients with normal renal function [28]. Of note, in the MM-010 study, patients with creatinine clearance <45 mL/min were excluded. Additional adverse events such as myalgias (16%) and skin rash (<10%) were less frequently seen with pomalidomide than with lenalidomide [29]. Similar to thalidomide and lenalidomide is the risk of VTE. Patients on pomalidomide should receive prophylaxis with, e.g., aspirin to minimize risk of these events.

5.5   Proteasome Inhibitors

5.5.1   Bortezomib

Bortezomib is a peptide boronic acid that reversibly and potently binds to the chymotrypsin-like $\beta5$ subunit of the proteasome 20S subunit [30, 31]. Inhibition of the proteasome by bortezomib in cell culture leads to apoptosis across multiple types of cancer cell lines. The effectiveness of bortezomib is particularly profound in MM, where MM cells typically produce large amounts of monoclonal immuno-globulin, a defining characteristic of this malignancy. In MM cells, treatment with bortezomib results in the accumulation of unfolded proteins, activating the unfolded protein response and subsequent cell cycle arrest [32]. Early clinical trials across different tumor types showed that bortezomib was unusually active in MM [33]. The SUMMIT trial was a phase II trial that evaluated bortezomib as single agent in patients with refractory disease [34]. Bortezomib was given 1.3 mg/m^2 intravenously (IV) on days 1, 4, 8, and 11 of 21-day cycle. In patients with a suboptimal response, dexamethasone 20 mg on the day of and day after bortezomib was added. The median number of prior therapies was six. As a single agent, the ORR was 27%. A phase III trial, the APEX trial, demonstrated higher response rates (ORR 38% vs. 18%, $p < 0.001$) and superior overall survival (1 year OS 80% vs. 66%, $p = 0.003$) with single-agent bortezomib compared to high-dose dexamethasone in patients who relapsed after 1–3 prior lines of treatment [19]. Based on the results of the SUMMIT trial, the FDA approved bortezomib for use in relapsed myeloma in 2003.

Peripheral neuropathy is the principal side effect of bortezomib. In the initial SUMMIT and CREST phase II trials of bortezomib in patients with relapsed MM, peripheral neuropathy occurred in 35% of patients, including 13% where it was grade ≥3 [35]. Dose reductions occurred in 12% of patients, and 5% of patients discontinued therapy because of neuropathy. Generally, the peripheral neuropathy is reversible. In the APEX study, 64% of patients had improvement or resolution to baseline at a median of 110 days, and the reversibility was higher when dose modifications were used. The effectiveness of bortezomib did not appear to be affected by these dose modifications.

A major change in treatment practice has been the shift from giving bortezomib IV (in the manner it was originally studied) to subcutaneously (SC). This was motivated by a randomized study of IV vs. SC administration in 222 patients with relapsed disease after 1–3 prior lines of treatment [36]. Patients received bortezomib according to the standard 21-day schedule, as a single agent. Peripheral neuropathy was significantly less common with the SC route, with grade ≥3 or more neuropathy of 6% compared to 12% ($p = 0.026$) with the standard IV route. The ORR was the same in both groups, 42%. An updated analysis of the trial showed comparable outcomes between the two routes [37]. Pharmacokinetic studies showed that systemic exposure was equivalent with either route, though the peak drug concentration was lower with the SC route [38]. Given the remarkably improved tolerability of the SC route with similar efficacy, the SC route is now approved by the FDA and now widely used.

Thrombocytopenia is the most common grade 3–4 adverse events with bortezomib. In the APEX trial, it occurred in 30% of patients. However, unlike the thrombocytopenia seen in traditional cytotoxic chemotherapy, the thrombocytopenia with bortezomib may be due to reversible effects on megakaryocyte function rather than direct cytotoxicity and is not cumulative [39]. Bortezomib is also associated with a significantly increased risk of herpes zoster. In the APEX trial, the incidence of herpes zoster was 13% compared to 5% ($p = 0.0002$) [40]. The use of acyclovir or equivalent for prophylaxis of this infection is standard practice [41].

In addition to changes in the route of administration, there is also an increasing use of weekly bortezomib, motivated by weekly schedules in the up-front setting [42, 43] that showed similar efficacy and improved tolerability. Consequently, over time, the practice has shifted from the twice/week, IV, 21-day schedule to increasing use of weekly bortezomib given SC (e.g., on days 1, 8, 15, 22 on a 35-day schedule), though many of the phase III trials using bortezomib follow the conventional 21-day schedule. Combinations with bortezomib are routinely used in the relapsed setting, as discussed below.

5.5.2 Carfilzomib

Carfilzomib is a second-generation PI. It is an epoxyketone that irreversibly binds to the proteasome through a covalent bond. Furthermore, compared with bortezomib, it has greater selectivity for chymotrypsin-like protease $\beta5$ subunit and lower affinity for trypsin- and caspase-like proteases [31]. These characteristics are in contrast to bortezomib, where proteasome binding is reversible and where bortezomib also inhibits other serine proteases (and which may account for its neurotoxicity) [44]. A phase II trial, PX-171-003, studied single-agent carfilzomib in heavily pretreated MM patients [45]. Carfilzomib was given as a single agent as an infusion at 20 mg/m^2 on days 1, 2, 8, 9, 15, and 16 of a 28-day cycle; with cycle 2, the dose was increased to 27 mg/m^2. The patients in this trial received a median of five prior lines of treatment, and the regimen showed an ORR of 23.7%. Based on the findings of this study, the FDA approved carfilzomib in July 2012 for patients with relapsed disease and who received at least two prior therapies, including bortezomib and an IMiD (e.g., lenalidomide) [46].

Unlike bortezomib, treatment-emergent peripheral neuropathy was markedly less common and severe, with grade 3–4 neuropathy occurring in 1.1% of patients. However, toxicities unique to carfilzomib included cardiac failure in 7% of patients. Dyspnea was reported in 35% of patients, including 5% experiencing grade 3 dyspnea. In our practice, we have found that lengthening the infusion time from the initially described 2–10 min infusion to, e.g., 30 min has decreased the rate of some of these side effects.

In patients progressing on a bortezomib-based regimen, a phase I–II trial found that replacing bortezomib with carfilzomib was safe and effective [47]. This replacement strategy was tested across multiple regimens, including carfilzomib and dexamethasone, carfilzomib with pegylated liposomal doxorubicin, and carfilzomib with cyclophosphamide and ascorbic acid. The ORR across this heterogeneous population was 43.2%, showing that the substitution of bortezomib with carfilzomib can recover responses in bortezomib-refractory disease.

5.5.2.1 ENDEAVOR

Recently, the ENDEAVOR trial directly compared carfilzomib with bortezomib in patients with relapsed disease [13]. This phase III study randomized patients with 1–3 prior lines of treatment to the combination of carfilzomib and dexamethasone or bortezomib and dexamethasone. Carfilzomib was given on days 1, 2, 8, 9, 15, and 16 with dexamethasone 20 mg on the days of carfilzomib plus days 22 and 23 on a 28-day cycle. The dosing of carfilzomib was higher than the initial studies, starting with 20 mg/m^2 on days 1 and 2 of cycle 1 and then increasing to 56 mg/m^2 there-after. Bortezomib was given according to the traditional schedule of 1.3 mg/m^2 on days 1, 4, 8, and 11 on a 21-day cycle with dexamethasone 20 mg the day of bortezomib and the day after. Bortezomib was given either IV or SC according to the investigator; most patients (79%) received SC bortezomib throughout the study. The ORR was significantly higher in the carfilzomib arm, 77% vs. 63% in the bortezomib arm ($p < 0.0001$), and median PFS was also higher, 18.7 months vs. 9.4 months ($p < 0.0001$). Of note, while 54% of patients had prior bortezomib, in a subgroup analysis, patients who were bortezomib naïve also showed significantly improved PFS in the carfilzomib arm.

Grade 2 or higher peripheral neuropathy was significantly higher in the bortezomib group compared to the carfilzomib group, 32% vs. 6%, respectively; grade 3 or higher peripheral neuropathy was 8% vs. 2%. Dose reductions due to adverse events were more common in the bortezomib group (48%) than in the carfilzomib group (23%), which may have compromised the true efficacy of bortezomib. Even though the majority of the patients received bortezomib SC, peripheral neuropathy continued to be an ongoing finding, and the majority of the dose reductions in the bortezomib group (62%) were due to peripheral neuropathy.

Additional notable differences in toxicity between the two groups included incidence of renal dysfunction. Acute renal failure, all grades, was higher in the carfilzomib arm vs. the bortezomib arm, 8% vs. 5%; grade 3 or higher, 4% vs. 3%. Hypertension, grade 3 or higher, was seen in carfilzomib compared to bortezomib, 9% vs. 3%. Cardiac failure (which included cardiac failure, decreased ejection fraction, pulmonary edema), all grades, was higher in the carfilzomib group compared to the bortezomib group (8.2% vs. 2.9%); grade 3 or higher (4.8% vs. 1.8%). Of note, in a subset of patients where serial echocardiograms were performed, reduction in left ventricular fraction was not different between groups.

5.5.2.2 Weekly Carfilzomib

A practical limitation of carfilzomib treatment is the twice/week schedule, especially given that patients may be on therapy for a prolonged duration. The CHAMPION-1 trial evaluated the safety and efficacy of giving carfilzomib *weekly* [48]. This phase I/II trial enrolled patients with 1–3 prior lines of treatment. Carfilzomib was given as a 30-min infusion on days 1, 8, and 15 with dexamethasone 40 mg weekly on a 28-day cycle. All patients received carfilzomib 20 mg/m^2 on day 1; patients received 45, 56, 70, or 88 mg/m^2 with subsequent infusions. The 70 mg/m^2 dose level was determined to be the MTD. Grade 3 or higher adverse events were uncommon (most common, fatigue, 11%), and the ORR was 77% with a PFS of 12.6 months. Notably, cardiac adverse events were not seen with using higher doses of carfilzomib. The rate of grade ≥3 dyspnea was 5%, similar to previous studies. The weekly dosing schedule in the CHAMPION-1 trial (20/70) is being compared to the conventional twice/week schedule (20/27) in an ongoing phase III trial, ARROW (NCT02412878).

5.5.3 Ixazomib

Ixazomib (previously known as MLN9708) is a new, *oral*, PI where preclinical data demonstrated superior pharmacodynamics with a shorter dissociation half-life and anti-tumor activity compared to bortezomib [49]. In preclinical models, ixazomib had activity in bortezomib-resistant MM cells [50].

Two phase I trials examined weekly [51] vs. twice/week dosing [52] of ixazomib as a single agent in patients with relapsed/refractory disease. In weekly dosing, ixazomib was given on days 1, 8, and 15 of a 28 cycle, and the twice/week dosing was similar to bortezomib on a 21-day cycle. The MTD for the weekly dosing was determined to be 2.97 mg/m^2 and 2 mg/m^2 for twice/week schedule. Pharmacokinetic studies showed a long terminal half-life of 3.6 to 11.3 days, providing support for once/week dosing. In these parallel trials, only one case of grade 3 peripheral neuropathy out of 60 patients in the weekly dosing cohort was observed. Rash (any grade) was reported in 9% of weekly dosing and 40% of the twice/week dosing trials. The patients in both of these trials were heavily pretreated, with a median of four prior lines of treatment. The ORR for weekly ixazomib was 18% (and 27% at the MTD).

5.5.3.1 TOURMALINE-MM1
The TOURMALINE-MM1 study compared the combination of ixazomib with lenalidomide and dexamethasone (IRd) vs. lenalidomide and dexamethasone (Rd) in a phase III, double-blind, randomized study in 712 patients with relapsed disease and 1–3 prior lines of treatment [14]. Of note, this triplet combination had already been presented as a phase I/II trial in newly diagnosed patients, with an ORR of 92% [53]. The trial in relapsed patients excluded patients who were refractory to prior PI-based or lenalidomide-based treatment. The majority of patients (69%) had prior bortezomib treatment, and only 12% had prior lenalidomide treatment. The median PFS was significantly higher in the IRd arm, 20.6 vs. 14.7 months in the Rd. arm ($p = 0.012$). The ORR was higher with IRd 78.3% vs. 71.5% ($p = 0.035$) along with very good partial response rate (VGPR) or better rate of 48.1% vs. 39% ($p = 0.014$). The toxicity profile between both arms was generally similar, including peripheral neuropathy. However, rash was higher in the ixazomib arm vs. the control arm: all grades, 36% vs. 17%, and grade 3–4 rash, 5% vs. 2% in the control arm. As with other PIs, thrombocytopenia was also higher, all grades, 31% vs. 16%, and grade 3–4, 19% vs. 9%.

Based on the encouraging findings in the TOURMALINE-MM1 study, the FDA approved ixazomib in November 2015 as part of a combination with lenalidomide and dexamethasone in patients with relapsed disease who have received at least one prior therapy. This was an important advance as an all oral triplet combination for relapsed disease. As treatment duration becomes longer (especially given the tolerability and efficacy of treatment), convenience for patients will also become increasingly important, and the availability of a PI as an oral agent may be a determining factor.

5.5.4   Proteasome Inhibitors Under Development

Two PIs under development include oprozomib and marizomib. **Oprozomib** (ONX 0912) is an expoxyketone analogous to carfilzomib but can be administered orally. Based on promising preclinical activity [54], oprozomib has been evaluated as a single agent and in combination with lenalidomide and dexamethasone or in combination with pomalidomide and dexamethasone. For example, a phase Ib/II trial evaluated oprozomib with dexamethasone in patients with 1–5 prior lines of therapy [55]. While this combination showed an ORR of 41.7%, gastrointestinal adverse events were notable in this trial (and in other oprozomib trials), with grade 3 diarrhea (21%) and nausea (10%).

Marizomib (NPI-0052) is a natural lactone compound derived from the marine actinomycetes *Salinispora tropica* [31]. Compared to bortezomib and carfilzomib, marizomib is unique in that it irreversibly inhibits both the chymotrypsin-like β5 and the trypsin-like β2 subunits, and preclinical models show that marizomib has synergistic anti-MM activity with pomalidomide [56]. Marizomib is given IV. A phase I study evaluated the combination of marizomib with pomalidomide and dexamethasone in patients with two or more prior lines of treatment and who had received prior lenalidomide and bortezomib [57]. This study enrolled 20 patients who were heavily pretreated with a median of five prior lines of treatment and achieved an ORR of 64%; no DLTs were observed.

5.6   HDAC Inhibitors

Histone deacetylase (HDAC) inhibitors such as vorinostat and now panobinostat are an important new class of cancer therapeutics [58]. By increasing the acetylation of histones, HDAC inhibitors modulate the transcriptional profile of cells and affect nuclear events. There are also other *non*histone substrates of HDACs in the cytoplasm through which HDAC inhibitors have various effects, such as protein degradation (via the aggresome) and protein-protein interactions.

In multiple myeloma, preclinical work with myeloma cell lines showed that HDAC inhibition synergizes with bortezomib, leading to mitochondrial dysfunction and apoptosis [59, 60]. However, as single agents, HDAC inhibitors are not active in MM. Clinical work with HDAC inhibitors began with the pan-HDAC inhibitor, vorinostat. VANTAGE 088 was a phase III trial of vorinostat in combination with bortezomib compared to bortezomib alone on a 21-day schedule in relapsed/refractory MM with 1–3 prior lines of therapy [61]. While this study showed significant improvement in progression-free survival, the difference was only 0.8 months (7.63 vs. 6.83 months) and not clinically meaningful.

5.6.1   PANORAMA 1

Panobinostat (LBH589) is another oral pan-HDAC inhibitor. PANORAMA 1 was a phase III trial comparing panobinostat, bortezomib, and dexamethasone to bortezomib and dexamethasone in a similar patient population as VANTAGE 088 with 1–3 prior lines of therapy [17]. Patients with disease refractory to bortezomib were excluded. Panobinostat 20 mg was given on days 1, 3, 5, 8, 10, and 12, and bortezomib was given IV on a conventional 21-day schedule on days 1, 4, 8, and 11. This study enrolled 768 patients, and the median progression-free survival was significantly longer in the panobinostat arm, 11.99 months vs. 8.08 months in the control arm ($p < 0.0001$). ORR trended higher in the panobinostat arm, 60.7% vs. 54.6% ($p = 0.09$). However, similar to the VANTAGE 088 trial, there was more grade 3–4 diarrhea in the panobinostat arm (25%) than in the control arm (8%). Deaths due to other causes besides progressive disease were also higher than in the panobinostat arm (7% vs. 3%). Given some of these concerns, the FDA decided against accelerated approval of panobinostat as second-line therapy in November 2014.

Panobinostat was reevaluated in 2015 as *third*-line therapy. In a prespecified subgroup analysis of 193 patients who received prior treatment with both bortezomib and an IMiD and a median of two prior therapies, the benefit of panobinostat was significantly higher in this population. The median PFS was 10.6 months in the panobinostat arm vs. 5.8 months in the control arm, and the ORR was also higher, 59% vs. 41%, respectively. Given the larger benefit in this more challenging to treat patient population, the FDA gave panobinostat accelerated approval in February 2015 in patients who received at least two prior lines of therapy, including bortezomib and an IMiD [62]. However, there is a boxed warning for diarrhea and cardiac events and arrhythmias, given the association between panobinostat and QT prolongation.

The ideal way to partner therapies with panobinostat remains to be determined, giving that the field has moved to giving bortezomib weekly and SC (given the better tolerability of this schedule and to minimize risk of peripheral neuropathy) rather than twice/week IV as was originally studied in the PANORAMA 1 trial. Newer combination strategies and dosing schedules may enhance efficacy, improve tolerability, and decrease some of the toxicities such as diarrhea. The approval of panobinostat sets the stage for other combinations such as with RVD (e.g., NCT01965353) and with carfilzomib (NCT01549431) in relapsed disease.

5.6.2 HDAC Inhibitors Under Development

Selective inhibition of specific HDACs is under active investigation. HDAC6 regulates acetylation of α-tubulin and the aggresome degradation pathway, and myeloma cells are vulnerable to HDAC6 inhibition [63]. Selective inhibition of HDAC6 may have an improved side effect profile compared to the pan-HDAC inhibition from vorinostat or panobinostat. The HDAC6-specific inhibitor **ricolinostat** (ACY-1215) has been in phase I and II clinical trials in combination with bortezomib (NCT01323751), lenalidomide (NCT01583283), or pomalidomide (NCT01997840) [64]. For example, the combination of ricolinostat and lenalidomide and dexamethasone was evaluated in 38 patients with one or more prior lines of therapy [65]. A maximum tolerated dose of ricolinostat was not reached. Common grade 3–4 hematologic adverse events included neutropenia (34%), anemia (5%), and thrombocytopenia (5%). Non-hematologic grade 3–4 adverse events included fatigue (18%) and diarrhea (5%). The ORR was 55%, and in patients who were refractory to lenalidomide, the ORR was 25%; the median PFS was 20.7 months. Notably, the frequency of diarrhea was less than with panobinostat, suggesting a beneficial effect of selective HDAC6 inhibition and/or the combination with an immunomodulatory rather than a PI. These findings suggest that the addition of ricolinostat to a lenalidomide-dexamethasone backbone adds to the efficacy of treatment without significantly adding additional toxicity.

5.7 Combinations of Immunomodulatory Drugs and Proteasome Inhibitors

Regimens based on the combination of an IMiD and a PI are active and well tolerated, and they are routinely used throughout the different phases of MM therapy. This combination was motivated on preclinical data showing potentiation of proteasome inhibition with IMiDs [66]. The following are examples of combinations in routine use:

5.7.1 Lenalidomide, Bortezomib, and Dexamethasone (RVD)

A phase I trial studied the combination of lenalidomide given on days 1–14 with bortezomib given IV on a conventional 21-day schedule in patients with relapsed/refractory study [67]. Dexamethasone was added to patients who had progressive disease. This study demonstrated efficacy in patients previously treated with lenalidomide or bortezomib and a MTD of lenalidomide 15 mg and bortezomib 1 mg/m^2 in this patient population, with an ORR of 39% and a median time to progression of 7.7 months. A larger phase II study with up-front use of dexamethasone in addition to lenalidomide and bortezomib (RVD) showed a higher response rate, with an ORR of 64%, median PFS 9.5 months, and median OS 30 months [68]. Of note, in this trial, 53% had prior bortezomib treatment, and only 6% had prior lenalidomide; the median number of prior treatments was 2. The rate of grade 3 peripheral neuropathy (3%) was lower than previous trials with bortezomib, which may reflect the lower dose of bortezomib of 1 mg/m^2 or the concomitant dosing of dexamethasone.

In our practice, when we give RVD in the relapsed setting, we generally give bortezomib on a weekly schedule, SC, for 4 out of 5 weeks with lenalidomide 15 mg on days 1–21 and then 14 days off, with dexamethasone the day of and day after bortezomib (similar to the "RVD-lite" schedule for newly diagnosed, transplant-ineligible patients [69]). Other schedules, such as a 28-day schedule where bortezomib is given on days 1, 8, and 15 combined with a traditional lenalidomide schedule, are in use as well [70].

5.7.2 Carfilzomib, Lenalidomide, and Dexamethasone (KRd-ASPIRE Trial)

The **ASPIRE** trial was a phase III trial that examined the combination of carfilzomib with lenalidomide and dexamethasone (KRd) compared to lenalidomide and dexamethasone in relapsed MM [16]. Patients were eligible to participate if they received 1–3 prior lines of therapy. Prior lenalidomide and bortezomib treatment were permitted if there was no disease progression with these drugs; the majority of patients (80.2%) had not seen prior lenalidomide therapy. Carfilzomib was given on days 1, 2, 8, 9, 15, and 16 on a 28-day cycle, with 20 mg/m^2 on the first 2 days of cycle 1 and then increased to 27 mg/m^2 subsequently. From cycles 13–18, the second week of carfilzomib was omitted. After cycle 18, carfilzomib was discontinued. Lenalidomide was given 25 mg on days 1–21 with dexamethasone 40 mg weekly; the same schedule of lenalidomide and dexamethasone was given in the control group. The ORR was significantly higher in the carfilzomib arm compared to the control arm, 87.1% vs. 66.7% ($p < 0.001$), and similarly the carfilzomib arm had a higher complete response rate, 31.8% vs. 9.3%. The median progression-free survival was 26.3 vs. 17.6 months ($p = 0.001$). The depth and duration of response in the treatment arm were unprecedented (though the control group also had a high response rate), and serious adverse events were uncommon. However, grade 3–4 dyspnea (2.8%), hypertension (4.3%), and cardiac failure (3.8%) were higher in the carfilzomib group, showing a similar toxicity profile seen in, e.g., the ENDEAVOR trial.

5.7.3 Carfilzomib, Pomalidomide, and Dexamethasone (KPd)

A phase I study evaluated the combination of carfilzomib, pomalidomide, and dexamethasone in patients with disease refractory to prior lenalidomide treatment [71]. A total of 32 patients were enrolled; they had received a median of 6 prior lines of treatment (range 2–12), and 100% were refractory to lenalidomide, and 97% were refractory to bortezomib. The starting dose level for carfilzomib was 20 mg/m^2 for the first 2 days and then increased to 27 mg/m^2 on a conventional carfilzomib schedule; pomalidomide was 4 mg on days 1–21; and dexamethasone was given 40 mg weekly. The maximum tolerated dose was dose level 1, likely reflecting the extensive treatment history of this patient population. Toxicities included grade ≥3 anemia (19%), thrombocytopenia (22%), and neutropenia (44%). Grade ≥3 non-hematologic toxicities were not common but did include two pulmonary embolism events with one death and four cases of pneumonia with one death. The ORR was 50% with a median PFS of 7.2 months, which is notable given that all patients were refractory to lenalidomide and nearly all were refractory to bortezomib. This trial showed that this regimen showed significant activity in a heavily pretreated, double refractory cohort, with side effect profile typical for an IMiD and PI combination.

5.7.4 Pomalidomide, Bortezomib, and Dexamethasone (PVD)

The MM-005 study evaluated in a phase I study the combination of pomalidomide, bortezomib, and dexamethasone in patients who had 1–4 prior lines of treatment and ≥2 cycles of lenalidomide plus a PI [72]. Patients had to be refractory to lenalidomide but not refractory to bortezomib. Treatment was given on a 21-day cycle, with pomalidomide on days 1–14; bortezomib (IV or SC) on days 1, 4, 8, and 11; and dexamethasone 20 mg on day of and day after bortezomib. The study enrolled 34 patients. There were no dose-limiting toxicities at the maximum planned dose of pomalidomide 4 mg and bortezomib 1.3 mg/m^2. The ORR was 65% with two complete responses. There were more grade ≥ 3 toxicities with IV than SC bortezomib, including neutropenia (80% vs. 25%) and thrombocytopenia (40% vs. 17%).

The Mayo Clinic evaluated the same combination in a similar patient population, though prior PI treatment was not required and the regimen was on a 28-day schedule [73]: pomalidomide 4 mg on days 1–21 and bortezomib (IV or SC) given on days 1, 8, 15, and 22. The study enrolled 47 patients, with a median of two prior lines of treatment. In this trial, the ORR was 85% ($\geq$ VGPR 45%) with a median PFS of 10.7 months. Grade ≥ 3 hematologic toxicities included neutropenia (68%) and anemia (2%) and thrombocytopenia (2%). These trials suggest that the PVD combination is highly active in MM refractory to lenalidomide and that weekly administration is associated with less adverse events.

Finally, OPTIMISMM (MM-007) is an ongoing phase III study to evaluate the combination of pomalidomide, bortezomib, and dexamethasone vs. bortezomib and dexamethasone in patients with 1–3 prior lines of treatment. In this trial, the treatment is given over a 21-day schedule, and bortezomib was given IV initially but is now permitted to be given SC.

5.7.5   Pomalidomide, Ixazomib, and Dexamethasone

A phase I/II study evaluated the combination of pomalidomide, ixazomib, and dexamethasone [74]. Patients who had two or more lines of therapy and who were refractory to lenalidomide and PIs were eligible to participate. Pomalidomide 2–4 mg was given for 21 out of 28 days with ixazomib (2.3–4 mg) on days 1, 8, and 15, with weekly dexamethasone, on a 28-day schedule. The trial enrolled 22 patients with a median of three prior lines of treatment. At the time of this writing, the trial is at dose level 4 (4 mg of pomalidomide with 4 mg of ixazomib). Grade 3–4 hematologic toxicities were as expected with an IMiD and PI combination, with grade 3–4 neutropenia (41%) and thrombocytopenia (18%). Rash adverse events were mild with one grade 1 and one grade 2 event. The ORR was 55%, including an ORR of 50% in patients who were dual refractory to the combination of lenalidomide with a PI.

5.8   Elotuzumab

Monoclonal antibodies designed against cell surface proteins such as CD20 (rituximab) or HER2 (trastuzumab), cytokines such as VEGF (bevacizumab), and now immune checkpoints such as PD1 (e.g., pembrolizumab) have transformed oncology care and are routinely used across nearly all tumor types. Elotuzumab is the first approved monoclonal antibody for myeloma [15]. Specifically, elotuzumab is a humanized recombinant monoclonal IgG1 antibody that targets signaling lymphocyte activation molecule (SLAMF7), also known as CS1 (CD2-subset-1). SLAMF7 is a cell surface glycoprotein that is highly expressed on both normal and MM plasma cells and is also found to a lower extent, on lymphocytes such as natural killer (NK) cells; it is absent in other tissues and hematopoietic stem cells [75, 76]. Expression of

SLAMF7 is nearly universal in MM, irrespective of cytogenetic abnormalities and degree of disease progression. Elotuzumab is proposed to have several modes of action: flagging myeloma cells for recognition by NK cells (i.e., antibody-dependent cellular cytotoxicity of MM cells involving natural killer (NK) cells) and enhancement of NK cell activity against MM cells by binding to SLAMF7 found on NK cells [77].

5.8.1 ELOQUENT-2

As a single agent, elotuzumab does not show significant clinical activity [78]. However, when combined with lenalidomide and dexamethasone, a phase I/II trial in relapsed or refractory MM showed an ORR of 84% with a median progression-free survival of 29 months [79]. More recently, a phase III study, ELOQUENT-2, compared the combination of elotuzumab, lenalidomide, and dexamethasone to lenalidomide and dexamethasone in patients with relapsed disease [15]. Patients with one to three prior lines of therapy were eligible to participate. Of note, the trial limited enrollment of patients with prior lenalidomide treatment to 10%, and these patients had to previously demonstrate at least a partial response to lenalidomide. Elotuzumab 10 mg/kg was given weekly for the first two cycles and then every other week. Lenalidomide and dexamethasone were given according to a conventional 28-day schedule. This trial enrolled 646 patients with a median of two prior lines of therapy. A significant proportion had high-risk cytogenetics (32% with del(17p) and 9% with t(4;14)). The elotuzumab-containing arm had superior progression-free survival (19.4 vs. 14.9 months in the control group, hazard ratio 0.7, $p < 0.001$), and the ORR was also higher (79% vs. 66%, $p < 0.001$). Adverse effects were similar between both arms, except for infusion reactions with elotuzumab (10% grade 1–2). Taken together, ELOQUENT-2 is the first study to show the benefit of adding a monoclonal antibody to conventional treatment in MM. In November 2015, the FDA approved elotuzumab in combination with lenalidomide and dexamethasone in patients who have received one to three prior lines of treatment.

5.9 Daratumumab

Daratumumab is a human IgG1κ monoclonal antibody that targets CD38, a transmembrane glycoprotein expressed in high levels myeloma cells but also found at low levels on lymphoid and myeloid cells [80]. Daratumumab was initially approved by the FDA in November 2015 for relapsed disease after three or more prior lines of therapy or who are double refractory to a PI and an IMiD, based on the results of two phase II trials showing significant single-agent activity [81, 82].

Notably, the following year, in 2016, saw the presentation of two pivotal phase III trials evaluating combinations with daratumumab in earlier stages of relapse. The CASTOR study (MMY3004) randomized patients with relapsed disease after one or more prior lines of treatment to daratumumab with bortezomib given SC and dexamethasone (on a 21-day schedule) vs. a doublet of bortezomib and dexamethasone [11]. The ORR and PFS were significantly higher in the daratumumab arm, 82.9%

vs. 63.2% ($p < 0.001$) and not estimable vs. 7.2 months, respectively, with a HR of 0.39 ($p < 0.001$). The POLLUX study (MMY3003) randomized patients with one or more prior lines of therapy to daratumumab with lenalidomide and dexamethasone vs. a doublet of lenalidomide and dexamethasone [83]. Patients with prior lenalidomide exposure who did not have disease refractory to lenalidomide were permitted to enroll, though this group comprised a small proportion of the trial population, 18%. Similar to the CASTOR study, the daratumumab arm had significantly higher ORR and PFS, 93% vs. 76% ($p < 0.0001$) and not estimable vs. 18.4 months, respectively, with a HR of 0.37 ($p < 0.0001$). Moreover, in the POLLUX trial, 22.4% of patients in the daratumumab arm achieved absence of minimal residual disease (sensitivity of 1 tumor cell per 10^5 white blood cells) compared to 4.6% in the control arm. The most common significant adverse events with both of the daratumumab combinations were neutropenia, thrombocytopenia, and anemia. Infusion-related reactions occurred in 45.3–47.7% of patients receiving daratumumab and were mostly grade 1 or 2. Almost all reactions occurred during the first infusion.

Both the CASTOR and POLLUX trials showed unprecedented improvement in outcomes in relapsed disease with the addition of daratumumab to standard doublet regimens while preserving excellent tolerability. In particular, the POLLUX sets a new bar for depth of response with achievement of negative minimal residual disease in nearly a quarter of patients, which has not been previously described in the relapsed setting. These findings establish the use of daratumumab combination earlier in the course of the disease and led to the approval by the FDA in November 2016 for patients with disease relapse after one prior line of therapy.

5.9.1 Combinations with Cyclophosphamide

5.9.1.1 Cyclophosphamide, Bortezomib, and Dexamethasone (CyBorD)

The combination of cyclophosphamide, bortezomib, and dexamethasone (CyBorD or VCD) is a standard, commonly used regimen in newly diagnosed patients, with an ORR of 93–100% [43, 84]. In relapsed disease, the outcomes of 55 patients with a mean number of 3.3 prior lines of treatment who were treated with CyBorD were reported [85]. Cyclophosphamide was given 300 mg/m^2 orally weekly, and bortezomib was given weekly at various dosing schedules (the majority received 1.5 mg/m^2 IV weekly), with dexamethasone 40 mg orally weekly, on a 28-day cycle. The ORR was 71%, 26% had VGPR or better, and 13% had a complete response (CR). Of note, patients who were naïve to PIs had an ORR of 95% vs. 57% ($p = 0.004$) who had prior exposure. Grade 1 peripheral neuropathy occurred in 16%, and 2% were grade 2; no patients had grade 3 or worse peripheral neuropathy. Median PFS was 9.2 months; in PI-naïve patients, it was 14.8 vs. 5.2 months ($p = 0.002$) in PI-exposed patients.

5.9.1.2 Carfilzomib, Cyclophosphamide, and Dexamethasone (CCyD)

Carfilzomib has also been combined with cyclophosphamide and dexamethasone as a treatment regimen in a phase II study newly diagnosed patients who were not transplant eligible [86]. In this study, carfilzomib was given on a standard schedule on days 1, 2, 8, 9, 15, and 16 on a 28-day cycle at 20 mg/m^2 on days 1 and 2 of cycle 1 and then 36 mg/m^2 subsequently. Cyclophosphamide 300 mg/m^2 orally was given on days 1, 8, and 15, and dexamethasone 40 mg was given orally on days 1, 8, 15, and 22. This study found a high response rate with an ORR of 95% and 20% stringent CR. In this older, transplant-ineligible patient population, the adverse event rate was comparable to other regimens, with grade ≥3 neutropenia (20%) and anemia (11%) and cardiopulmonary adverse events (7%). This regimen is currently being evaluated in patients after one prior line of treatment and compared to CyBorD in the Myeloma UK five study [87]. In this study, the dosing is similar to the regimen in newly diagnosed patients, though cyclophosphamide is given at 500 mg. Preliminary toxicity data has been presented so far, with grade ≥3 hematologic adverse events including anemia (19.4%), neutropenia (12%), and thrombocytopenia (10.5%) and non-hematologic ≥ grade 3 including infections (20.9%).

5.10 Salvage Infusional Regimens

In select patients who are experiencing an aggressive, rapid relapse with, e.g., a high burden of extramedullary disease and where there is an urgent need for cytoreduction, a salvage infusional regimen combining traditional cytotoxic drugs may be appropriate. These regimens include DCEP (dexamethasone, cyclophosphamide, etoposide, cisplatin), VTD-PACE (bortezomib, thalidomide, dexamethasone, cisplatin, doxorubicin, cyclophosphamide, etoposide), and CVAD (dexamethasone, cyclophosphamide, vincristine, and doxorubicin). In some cases, these regimens may be used as a "bridge" to autologous stem cell transplant or to the next line of therapy. A retrospective analysis evaluated the use of these three infusional regimens in 107 patients who had received a median of three prior lines of treatment [88]. There was no difference in survival across these regimens, with an overall median PFS of 4.5 months and a median OS of 8.5 months across the entire cohort. Toxicities were significant, including febrile neutropenia (DCEP, 29%; VTD-PACE, 50%; and CVAD, 39%) and treatment-related mortality (DCEP, 6%, VTD-PACE 5%, and CVAD 9%).

5.10.1 Salvage Autologous Stem Cell Transplant

A salvage autologous stem cell transplant (SCT) may be considered as another treatment modality for patients in their first or second relapse. Prior to a salvage SCT, induction chemotherapy using e.g., a regimen described in this chapter is typically given. As a general rule of thumb, the PFS from a salvage SCT is generally half of that obtained from the initial transplant [89]. A retrospective study of 81 patients who received a salvage autologous SCT compared outcomes for patients who relapsed ≤24 months after their initial SCT vs. patients who had disease relapse >24 months [90]. The former group had a significantly worse PFS of 9.83 months and OS of 28.47 months, compared to the latter group with PFS of 17.3 months and OS of 71.3 months ($p < 0.05$ and $p = 0.006$, respectively). Similar findings were seen in a larger retrospective study of 187 patients: patients who underwent a salvage SCT ≥36 months after the initial SCT had the most benefit, with 3-year overall survival of 58% vs. 42% in patients who underwent a SCT <36 months [91]. In a smaller study of 30 patients who underwent salvage SCT, patients who underwent transplant <18 months after relapse from the initial transplant had a median progression-free survival of only 4.2 months [92]. Based on these findings, patients who relapse less than 18 months should consider reinduction chemotherapy rather than pursuing a salvage autologous SCT.

Furthermore, while an autologous SCT is an option for patients who have enjoyed a long time in remission prior to relapse, an ongoing question is whether or not high-dose treatment is superior to standard treatment. A retrospective study of 172 patients did not find a significant difference in event-free survival (1.3 vs. 0.9 years, $p = 0.73$) or overall survival (2.9 vs. 1.7 years, $p = 0.07$) in patients who received autologous SCT vs. conventional chemotherapy [93]. A phase III trial examined this question, the Myeloma X (Intensive) Trial, evaluating 297 patients who had relapsed 18 months after a previous autologous SCT and randomizing them to high-dose melphalan plus salvage autologous SCT vs. oral cyclophosphamide 400 mg/m^2/week for 12 weeks [94]. Prior to randomization, all patients received induction treatment with bortezomib, doxorubicin, and dexamethasone; 174 patients were ultimately randomized. The median time to progression was significantly longer in the ASCT group, 19 vs. 11 months ($p < 0.0001$). An updated analysis of the study showed an improvement in overall survival in the ASCT group, 67 vs. 52 months ($p = 0.022$) [95]. However, a significant limitation of the study is the use of oral cyclophosphamide, a regimen that is no longer commonly used with the availability of more effective treatments, suggesting that the difference between ASCT and conventional treatment may be less pronounced with more modern treatment regimens.

5.10.2 Allogeneic Stem Cell Transplant

In certain circumstances, allogeneic SCT is another option for patients at time of first or second relapse, especially fitter patients with high-risk features and who have a suitable donor. However, several older retrospective analyses comparing allogeneic transplant vs. autologous transplant suggest a higher non-relapse mortality rate and worse PFS and OS with the allogeneic approach [89, 96].

5.11 Choice of Treatment

As is true with the initial treatment, multiple factors play into the choice of treatment for relapsed disease. These include host factors, such as the performance status or frailty of the patient and disease-specific factors. A patient presenting with extramedullary disease or acute onset of hypercalcemia and renal dysfunction may warrant more aggressive treatment than a patient with a slowly rising monoclonal protein (who may be closely observed). The time of the relapse is also important too, as patients who relapse early, for example, less than a year after an autologous SCT (which occurs in 24% of patients undergoing autologous SCT), have a worse prognosis [97]. This finding continues to hold true when more novel induction treatment regimens are used, with patients with an early relapse having a median OS of 20 months following SCT compared to 93 months [98]. For patient with an early relapse, more aggressive treatment, e.g., with a triplet regimen, should be considered.

The prior treatment history also needs to be carefully reviewed to assess exposure history as well as toxicity to treatments, such as peripheral neuropathy. Significant cardiac disease should also be noted. The treatment schedule also may play a role, depending on the patient's ability to travel for treatment, which may be influenced by the patient's level of fitness and performance status. Related to the schedule is also convenience, e.g., the ability to self-administer ixazomib at home.

5.11.1 Retreatment

Conventionally, in oncology practice, retreatment with the same agent following progression is deferred given assumptions about drug resistance [99]. In MM, given its natural history of response followed by relapse, patients may need to be retreated with similar regimens over the course of their illness. The RETRIEVE study showed the efficacy of retreatment with bortezomib [100]. This prospective study enrolled 130 patients who relapsed 6 months or more after having achieved at least a partial response to bortezomib. The median time from prior bortezomib treatment was 13.9 months (range, 5–39 months). During retreatment, 28% of patients received bortezomib alone, and 72% received bortezomib with dexamethasone. Bortezomib was given IV according to the standard 21-day schedule. There were no grade 3 or higher neuropathy adverse events. The ORR was 40%, indicating that retreatment with bortezomib was effective. Similar findings were also seen in an updated analysis of the VISTA trial, which was a randomized trial comparing VMP (bortezomib, melphalan, and prednisone) to MP (melphalan and prednisone) in newly diagnosed patients who were not eligible for high-dose treatment [101]. In this study, for patients with relapsing disease where the treatment-free interval was ≤12 months, the response rate was 25% for bortezomib retreatment compared to 71% for patients where the treatment-free interval was >12 months.

Retreatment with IMiDs was examined in a retrospective study of 140 patients who received either thalidomide-dexamethasone or lenalidomide-dexamethasone for treatment of relapsed disease [102]. These patients had received a median of two prior lines of treatment, including a SCT in 75%. In patients who previously received lenalidomide, retreatment with lenalidomide had an ORR of 54%. In patients who discontinued first-line lenalidomide therapy because of disease progression, the ORR was 25%. Of note, retreatment with thalidomide had a lower response rate after prior lenalidomide (ORR 20%) or prior thalidomide (ORR 30%). This study indicates that patients who had disease progression with prior lenalidomide therapy can still achieve a response with retreatment with lenalidomide.

Conclusions

The treatment options for MM patients with relapsed disease have expanded remarkably in the past 4 years, with the FDA approval of carfilzomib in July 2012 followed by pomalidomide in February 2013, panobinostat in February 2015, and recently an unprecedented three approvals in November 2015: daratumumab, ixazomib, and elotuzumab. These new additions are effective with very manageable side effects, improving survival for patients and enhancing their quality of life. The field is also moving toward more active and equally important, well-tolerated, three-drug combinations. Ongoing studies will better define the sequence and the components of these regimens.

References

1. Kumar SK, Rajkumar SV, Dispenzieri A, Lacy MQ, Hayman SR, Buadi FK, Zeldenrust SR, Dingli D, Russell SJ, Lust JA, et al. Improved survival in multiple myeloma and the impact of novel therapies. Blood. 2008b;111:2516–20.
2. Rajkumar SV, Harousseau JL, Durie B, Anderson KC, Dimopoulos M, Kyle R, Blade J, Richardson P, Orlowski R, Siegel D, et al. Consensus recommendations for the uniform reporting of clinical trials: report of the International Myeloma Workshop Consensus Panel 1. Blood. 2011;117:4691–5.
3. Rajkumar SV, Richardson P, San Miguel JF. Guidelines for determination of the number of prior lines of therapy in multiple myeloma. Blood. 2015;126:921–2.
4. Durie BG, Harousseau JL, Miguel JS, Blade J, Barlogie B, Anderson K, Gertz M, Dimopoulos M, Westin J, Sonneveld P, et al. International uniform response criteria for multiple myeloma. Leukemia. 2006;20:1467–73.
5. Fernandez de Larrea C, Jimenez R, Rosinol L, Gine E, Tovar N, Cibeira MT, Fernandez-Aviles F, Martinez C, Rovira M, Blade J. Pattern of relapse and progression after autologous SCT as upfront treatment for multiple myeloma. Bone Marrow Transplant. 2014;49:223–7.
6. Kronke J, Udeshi ND, Narla A, Grauman P, Hurst SN, McConkey M, Svinkina T, Heckl D, Comer E, Li X, et al. Lenalidomide causes selective degradation of IKZF1 and IKZF3 in multiple myeloma cells. Science. 2014;343:301–5.
7. Lopez-Girona A, Mendy D, Ito T, Miller K, Gandhi AK, Kang J, Karasawa S, Carmel G, Jackson P, Abbasian M, et al. Cereblon is a direct protein target for immunomodulatory and antiproliferative activities of lenalidomide and pomalidomide. Leukemia. 2012;26:2326–35.
8. Lu G, Middleton RE, Sun H, Naniong M, Ott CJ, Mitsiades CS, Wong KK, Bradner JE, Kaelin WG Jr. The myeloma drug lenalidomide promotes the cereblon-dependent destruction of Ikaros proteins. Science. 2014;343:305–9.
9. Weber DM, Chen C, Niesvizky R, Wang M, Belch A, Stadtmauer EA, Siegel D, Borrello I, Rajkumar SV, Chanan-Khan AA, et al. Lenalidomide plus dexamethasone for relapsed multiple myeloma in North America. N Engl J Med. 2007;357:2133–42.
10. Dimopoulos M, Spencer A, Attal M, Prince HM, Harousseau JL, Dmoszynska A, San Miguel J, Hellmann A, Facon T, Foa R, et al. Lenalidomide plus dexamethasone for relapsed or refractory multiple myeloma. N Engl J Med. 2007;357:2123–32.

11. Palumbo A, Chanan-Khan A, Weisel K, Nooka AK, Masszi T, Beksac M, Spicka I, Hungria V, Munder M, Mateos MV, et al. Daratumumab, bortezomib, and dexamethasone for multiple myeloma. N Engl J Med. 2016;375:754–66.
12. Dimopoulos MA, Oriol A, Nahi H, San-Miguel J, Bahlis NJ, Usmani SZ, Rabin N, Orlowski RZ, Komarnicki M, Suzuki K, et al. Daratumumab, lenalidomide, and dexamethasone for multiple myeloma. N Engl J Med. 2016c;375:1319–31.
13. Dimopoulos MA, Moreau P, Palumbo A, Joshua D, Pour L, Hajek R, Facon T, Ludwig H, Oriol A, Goldschmidt H, et al. Carfilzomib and dexamethasone versus bortezomib and dexamethasone for patients with relapsed or refractory multiple myeloma (ENDEAVOR): a randomised, phase 3, open-label, multicentre study. Lancet Oncol. 2016a;17:27–38.
14. Moreau P, Masszi T, Grzasko N, Bahlis NJ, Hansson M, Pour L, Sandhu I, Ganly P, Baker BW, Jackson S, et al. Ixazomib, an investigational oral proteasome inhibitor (PI), in combination with lenalidomide and dexamethasone (IRd), significantly extends progression-free survival (PFS) for patients (Pts) with relapsed and/or refractory multiple myeloma (RRMM): the phase 3 tourmaline-MM1 study (NCT01564537). Blood. 2015;126:727.
15. Lonial S, Dimopoulos M, Palumbo A, White D, Grosicki S, Spicka I, Walter-Croneck A, Moreau P, Mateos MV, Magen H, et al. Elotuzumab therapy for relapsed or refractory multiple myeloma. N Engl J Med. 2015;373:621–31.
16. Stewart AK, Rajkumar SV, Dimopoulos MA, Masszi T, Spicka I, Oriol A, Hajek R, Rosinol L, Siegel DS, Mihaylov GG, et al. Carfilzomib, lenalidomide, and dexamethasone for relapsed multiple myeloma. N Engl J Med. 2015;372:142–52.
17. San-Miguel JF, Hungria VT, Yoon SS, Beksac M, Dimopoulos MA, Elghandour A, Jedrzejczak WW, Gunther A, Nakorn TN, Siritanaratkul N, et al. Panobinostat plus bortezomib and dexamethasone versus placebo plus bortezomib and dexamethasone in patients with relapsed or relapsed and refractory multiple myeloma: a multicentre, randomised, double-blind phase 3 trial. Lancet Oncol. 2014;15:1195–206.
18. San Miguel J, Weisel K, Moreau P, Lacy M, Song K, Delforge M, Karlin L, Goldschmidt H, Banos A, Oriol A, et al. Pomalidomide plus low-dose dexamethasone versus high-dose dexamethasone alone for patients with relapsed and refractory multiple myeloma (MM-003): a randomised, open-label, phase 3 trial. Lancet Oncol. 2013;14:1055–66.
19. Richardson PG, Sonneveld P, Schuster MW, Irwin D, Stadtmauer EA, Facon T, Harousseau JL, Ben-Yehuda D, Lonial S, Goldschmidt H, et al. Bortezomib or high-dose dexamethasone for relapsed multiple myeloma. N Engl J Med. 2005;352:2487–98.
20. Dimopoulos MA, Chen C, Spencer A, Niesvizky R, Attal M, Stadtmauer EA, Petrucci MT, Yu Z, Olesnyckyj M, Zeldis JB, et al. Long-term follow-up on overall survival from the MM-009 and MM-010 phase III trials of lenalidomide plus dexamethasone in patients with relapsed or refractory multiple myeloma. Leukemia. 2009;23:2147–52.
21. Palumbo A, Rajkumar SV, Dimopoulos MA, Richardson PG, San Miguel J, Barlogie B, Harousseau J, Zonder JA, Cavo M, Zangari M, et al. Prevention of thalidomide- and lenalidomide-associated thrombosis in myeloma. Leukemia. 2008;22:414–23.
22. Zonder JA, Barlogie B, Durie BG, McCoy J, Crowley J, Hussein MA. Thrombotic complications in patients with newly diagnosed multiple myeloma treated with lenalidomide and dexamethasone: benefit of aspirin prophylaxis. Blood. 2006;108:403.
23. Rajkumar SV, Jacobus S, Callander NS, Fonseca R, Vesole DH, Williams ME, Abonour R, Siegel DS, Katz M, Greipp PR, et al. Lenalidomide plus high-dose dexamethasone versus lenalidomide plus low-dose dexamethasone as initial therapy for newly diagnosed multiple myeloma: an open-label randomised controlled trial. Lancet Oncol. 2010;11:29–37.
24. Palumbo A, Bringhen S, Kumar SK, Lupparelli G, Usmani S, Waage A, Larocca A, van der Holt B, Musto P, Offidani M, et al. Second primary malignancies with lenalidomide therapy for newly diagnosed myeloma: a meta-analysis of individual patient data. Lancet Oncol. 2014;15:333–42.
25. Richardson PG, Siegel DS, Vij R, Hofmeister CC, Baz R, Jagannath S, Chen C, Lonial S, Jakubowiak A, Bahlis N, et al. Pomalidomide alone or in combination with low-dose dexamethasone in relapsed and refractory multiple myeloma: a randomized phase 2 study. Blood. 2014c;123:1826–32.

26. Morgan G, Palumbo A, Dhanasiri S, Lee D, Weisel K, Facon T, Delforge M, Oriol A, Zaki M, Yu X, et al. Overall survival of relapsed and refractory multiple myeloma patients after adjusting for crossover in the MM-003 trial for pomalidomide plus low-dose dexamethasone. Br J Haematol. 2015;168:820–3.

27. Hoffmann M, Kasserra C, Reyes J, Schafer P, Kosek J, Capone L, Parton A, Kim-Kang H, Surapaneni S, Kumar G. Absorption, metabolism and excretion of [14C]pomalidomide in humans following oral administration. Cancer Chemother Pharmacol. 2013;71:489–501.

28. Weisel K, Dimopoulos MA, Cavo M, Ocio EM, Palumbo A, Corradini P, Delforge M, Oriol A, Goldschmidt H, Conticello C, et al. Pomalidomide + low-dose dexamethasone in patients with refractory or relapsed and refractory multiple myeloma and renal impairment: analysis of patients from the phase 3b stratus trial (MM-010). Blood. 2014;124:4755.

29. Dimopoulos MA, Leleu X, Palumbo A, Moreau P, Delforge M, Cavo M, Ludwig H, Morgan GJ, Davies FE, Sonneveld P, et al. Expert panel consensus statement on the optimal use of pomalidomide in relapsed and refractory multiple myeloma. Leukemia. 2014;28:1573–85.

30. Adams J. The development of proteasome inhibitors as anticancer drugs. Cancer Cell. 2004;5:417–21.

31. Moreau P, Richardson PG, Cavo M, Orlowski RZ, San Miguel JF, Palumbo A, Harousseau JL. Proteasome inhibitors in multiple myeloma: 10 years later. Blood. 2012b;120:947–59.

32. Obeng EA, Carlson LM, Gutman DM, Harrington WJ Jr, Lee KP, Boise LH. Proteasome inhibitors induce a terminal unfolded protein response in multiple myeloma cells. Blood. 2006;107:4907–16.

33. Orlowski RZ, Stinchcombe TE, Mitchell BS, Shea TC, Baldwin AS, Stahl S, Adams J, Esseltine DL, Elliott PJ, Pien CS, et al. Phase I trial of the proteasome inhibitor PS-341 in patients with refractory hematologic malignancies. J Clin Oncol. 2002;20:4420–7.

34. Richardson PG, Barlogie B, Berenson J, Singhal S, Jagannath S, Irwin D, Rajkumar SV, Srkalovic G, Alsina M, Alexanian R, et al. A phase 2 study of bortezomib in relapsed, refractory myeloma. N Engl J Med. 2003;348:2609–17.

35. Richardson PG, Briemberg H, Jagannath S, Wen PY, Barlogie B, Berenson J, Singhal S, Siegel DS, Irwin D, Schuster M, et al. Frequency, characteristics, and reversibility of peripheral neuropathy during treatment of advanced multiple myeloma with bortezomib. J Clin Oncol. 2006;24:3113–20.

36. Moreau P, Pylypenko H, Grosicki S, Karamanesht I, Leleu X, Grishunina M, Rekhtman G, Masliak Z, Robak T, Shubina A, et al. Subcutaneous versus intravenous administration of bortezomib in patients with relapsed multiple myeloma: a randomised, phase 3, non-inferiority study. Lancet Oncol. 2010;12:431–40.

37. Arnulf B, Pylypenko H, Grosicki S, Karamanesht I, Leleu X, van de Velde H, Feng H, Cakana A, Deraedt W, Moreau P. Updated survival analysis of a randomized phase III study of subcutaneous versus intravenous bortezomib in patients with relapsed multiple myeloma. Haematologica. 2012;97:1925–8.

38. Moreau P, Karamanesht II, Domnikova N, Kyselyova MY, Vilchevska KV, Doronin VA, Schmidt A, Hulin C, Leleu X, Esseltine DL, et al. Pharmacokinetic, pharmacodynamic and covariate analysis of subcutaneous versus intravenous administration of bortezomib in patients with relapsed multiple myeloma. Clin Pharmacokinet. 2012a;51:823–9.

39. Lonial S, Waller EK, Richardson PG, Jagannath S, Orlowski RZ, Giver CR, Jaye DL, Francis D, Giusti S, Torre C, et al. Risk factors and kinetics of thrombocytopenia associated with bortezomib for relapsed, refractory multiple myeloma. Blood. 2005;106:3777–84.

40. Chanan-Khan A, Sonneveld P, Schuster MW, Stadtmauer EA, Facon T, Harousseau JL, Ben-Yehuda D, Lonial S, Goldschmidt H, Reece D, et al. Analysis of herpes zoster events among bortezomib-treated patients in the phase III APEX study. J Clin Oncol. 2008;26:4784–90.

41. Vickrey E, Allen S, Mehta J, Singhal S. Acyclovir to prevent reactivation of varicella zoster virus (herpes zoster) in multiple myeloma patients receiving bortezomib therapy. Cancer. 2009;115:229–32.

42. Girnius SK, Lee S, Kambhampati S, Rose MG, Mohiuddin A, Houranieh A, Zimelman A, Grady T, Mehta P, Behler C, et al. A phase II trial of weekly bortezomib and dexamethasone in veterans with newly diagnosed multiple myeloma not eligible for or who deferred autologous stem cell transplantation. Br J Haematol. 2015;169:36–43.

43. Reeder CB, Reece DE, Kukreti V, Chen C, Trudel S, Laumann K, Hentz J, Pirooz NA, Piza JG, Tiedemann R, et al. Once- versus twice-weekly bortezomib induction therapy with CyBorD in newly diagnosed multiple myeloma. Blood. 2010;115:3416–7.

44. Arastu-Kapur S, Anderl JL, Kraus M, Parlati F, Shenk KD, Lee SJ, Muchamuel T, Bennett MK, Driessen C, Ball AJ, et al. Nonproteasomal targets of the proteasome inhibitors bortezomib and carfilzomib: a link to clinical adverse events. Clin Cancer Res. 2011;17: 2734–43.

45. Siegel DS, Martin T, Wang M, Vij R, Jakubowiak AJ, Lonial S, Trudel S, Kukreti V, Bahlis N, Alsina M, et al. A phase 2 study of single-agent carfilzomib (PX-171-003-A1) in patients with relapsed and refractory multiple myeloma. Blood. 2012;120:2817–25.

46. Herndon TM, Deisseroth A, Kaminskas E, Kane RC, Koti KM, Rothmann MD, Habtemariam B, Bullock J, Bray JD, Hawes J, et al. U.S. Food and Drug Administration Approval: carfilzomib for the treatment of multiple myeloma. Clin Cancer Res. 2013;19:4559–63.

47. Berenson JR, Hilger JD, Yellin O, Dichmann R, Patel-Donnelly D, Boccia RV, Bessudo A, Stampleman L, Gravenor D, Eshaghian S, et al. Replacement of bortezomib with carfilzomib for multiple myeloma patients progressing from bortezomib combination therapy. Leukemia. 2014;28:1529–36.

48. Berenson J, Cartmell A, Lyons R, Harb W, Tzachanis D, Agajanian R, Boccia RV, Coleman M, Moss RA, Rifkin RM, et al. Weekly carfilzomib with dexamethasone for patients with relapsed or refractory multiple myeloma: updated results from the phase 1/2 study champion-1 (NCT01677858). Blood. 2015;126:373.

49. Kupperman E, Lee EC, Cao Y, Bannerman B, Fitzgerald M, Berger A, Yu J, Yang Y, Hales P, Bruzzese F, et al. Evaluation of the proteasome inhibitor MLN9708 in preclinical models of human cancer. Cancer Res. 2010;70:1970–80.

50. Chauhan D, Tian Z, Zhou B, Kuhn D, Orlowski R, Raje N, Richardson P, Anderson KC. In vitro and in vivo selective antitumor activity of a novel orally bioavailable proteasome inhibitor MLN9708 against multiple myeloma cells. Clin Cancer Res. 2011;17:5311–21.

51. Kumar SK, Bensinger WI, Zimmerman TM, Reeder CB, Berenson JR, Berg D, Hui AM, Gupta N, Di Bacco A, Yu J, et al. Phase 1 study of weekly dosing with the investigational oral proteasome inhibitor ixazomib in relapsed/refractory multiple myeloma. Blood. 2014a;124:1047–55.

52. Richardson PG, Baz R, Wang M, Jakubowiak AJ, Laubach JP, Harvey RD, Talpaz M, Berg D, Liu G, Yu J, et al. Phase 1 study of twice-weekly ixazomib, an oral proteasome inhibitor, in relapsed/refractory multiple myeloma patients. Blood. 2014a;124:1038–46.

53. Kumar SK, Berdeja JG, Niesvizky R, Lonial S, Laubach JP, Hamadani M, Stewart AK, Hari P, Roy V, Vescio R, et al. Safety and tolerability of ixazomib, an oral proteasome inhibitor, in combination with lenalidomide and dexamethasone in patients with previously untreated multiple myeloma: an open-label phase 1/2 study. Lancet Oncol. 2014b;15: 1503–12.

54. Shah J, Niesvizky R, Stadtmauer E, Rifkin RM, Berenson J, Berdeja JG, Sharman JP, Lyons R, Klippel Z, Wong H, et al. Oprozomib, pomalidomide, and dexamethasone (OPomd) in patients (Pts) with relapsed and/or refractory multiple myeloma (RRMM): initial results of a phase 1b study (NCT01999335). Blood. 2015a;126:378.

55. Hari PN, Shain KH, Voorhees PM, Gabrail N, Abidi MH, Zonder J, Boccia RV, Richardson PG, Neuman LL, Dixon SJ, et al. Oprozomib and dexamethasone in patients with relapsed and/or refractory multiple myeloma: initial results from the dose escalation portion of a phase 1b/2, multicenter, open-label study. Blood. 2014;124:3453.

56. Das DS, Ray A, Song Y, Richardson P, Trikha M, Chauhan D, Anderson KC. Synergistic anti-myeloma activity of the proteasome inhibitor marizomib and the IMiD((R)) immunomodulatory drug pomalidomide. Br J Haematol. 2015;171:798–812.

57. Spencer A, Laubach JP, Zonder JA, Badros AZ, Harrison S, Khot A, Chauhan D, Anderson KC, Reich SD, Trikha M, et al. Phase 1, multicenter, open-label, combination study (NPI-0052-107; NCT02103335) of pomalidomide (POM), marizomib (MRZ, NPI-0052), and low-dose dexamethasone (LD-DEX) in patients with relapsed and refractory multiple myeloma. Blood. 2015;126:4220.

58. Minucci S, Pelicci PG. Histone deacetylase inhibitors and the promise of epigenetic (and more) treatments for cancer. Nat Rev Cancer. 2006;6:38–51.
59. Pei XY, Dai Y, Grant S. Synergistic induction of oxidative injury and apoptosis in human multiple myeloma cells by the proteasome inhibitor bortezomib and histone deacetylase inhibitors. Clin Cancer Res. 2004;10:3839–52.
60. Richardson PG, Mitsiades CS, Laubach JP, Hajek R, Spicka I, Dimopoulos MA, Moreau P, Siegel DS, Jagannath S, Anderson KC. Preclinical data and early clinical experience supporting the use of histone deacetylase inhibitors in multiple myeloma. Leuk Res. 2013;37:829–37.
61. Dimopoulos M, Siegel DS, Lonial S, Qi J, Hajek R, Facon T, Rosinol L, Williams C, Blacklock H, Goldschmidt H, et al. Vorinostat or placebo in combination with bortezomib in patients with multiple myeloma (VANTAGE 088): a multicentre, randomised, double-blind study. Lancet Oncol. 2013;14:1129–40.
62. FDA. FDA approves Farydak for treatment of multiple myeloma. 2015.
63. Hideshima T, Bradner JE, Wong J, Chauhan D, Richardson P, Schreiber SL, Anderson KC. Small-molecule inhibition of proteasome and aggresome function induces synergistic antitumor activity in multiple myeloma. Proc Natl Acad Sci U S A. 2005;102:8567–72.
64. Raje NS, Bensinger W, Cole CE, Lonial S, Jagannath S, Arce-Lara CE, Valent J, Rosko AE, Harb WA, Sandhu I, et al. Ricolinostat (ACY-1215), the first selective HDAC6 inhibitor, combines safely with pomalidomide and dexamethasone and shows promising early results in relapsed-and-refractory myeloma (ACE-MM-102 study). Blood. 2015;126:4228.
65. Yee AJ, Bensinger WI, Supko JG, Voorhees PM, Berdeja JG, Richardson PG, Libby EN, Wallace EE, Birrer NE, Burke JN, et al. Ricolinostat plus lenalidomide, and dexamethasone in relapsed or refractory multiple myeloma: a multicentre phase 1b trial. Lancet Oncol. 2016;17:1569–78.
66. Mitsiades N, Mitsiades CS, Poulaki V, Chauhan D, Richardson PG, Hideshima T, Munshi NC, Treon SP, Anderson KC. Apoptotic signaling induced by immunomodulatory thalidomide analogs in human multiple myeloma cells: therapeutic implications. Blood. 2002;99:4525–30.
67. Richardson PG, Weller E, Jagannath S, Avigan DE, Alsina M, Schlossman RL, Mazumder A, Munshi NC, Ghobrial IM, Doss D, et al. Multicenter, phase I, dose-escalation trial of lenalidomide plus bortezomib for relapsed and relapsed/refractory multiple myeloma. J Clin Oncol. 2009;27:5713–9.
68. Richardson PG, Xie W, Jagannath S, Jakubowiak A, Lonial S, Raje NS, Alsina M, Ghobrial IM, Schlossman RL, Munshi NC, et al. A phase 2 trial of lenalidomide, bortezomib, and dexamethasone in patients with relapsed and relapsed/refractory myeloma. Blood. 2014d;123:1461–9.
69. O'Donnell EK, Laubach JP, Yee AJ, Huff CA, Basile FG, Wade PM, Paba-Prada CE, Ghobrial IM, Schlossman RL, Couture NR, et al. A phase II study of modified lenalidomide, bortezomib, and dexamethasone (RVD-lite) for transplant-ineligible patients with newly diagnosed multiple myeloma. Blood. 2015;126:4217.
70. Broijl, A., Kersten, M.J., Alemayehu, W.G., Levin, M.D., de Weerdt, O., Vellenga, E., Meijer, E., Wittebol, S., Tanis, B.C., Cornelisse, P.B., et al. (2015). Phase I/II trial of weekly bortezomib with lenalidomide and dexamethasone in first relapse or primary refractory myeloma. Haematologica. 101(4): e149–e152.
71. Shah JJ, Stadtmauer EA, Abonour R, Cohen AD, Bensinger WI, Gasparetto C, Kaufman JL, Lentzsch S, Vogl DT, Gomes CL, et al. Carfilzomib, pomalidomide, and dexamethasone for relapsed or refractory myeloma. Blood. 2015b;126:2284–90.
72. Richardson PG, Hofmeister C, Raje NS, Siegel D, Lonial S, Laubach JP, Efebera YA, Vesole DH, Nooka AK, Rosenblatt J, et al. A phase 1, multicenter study of pomalidomide, bortezomib, and low-dose dexamethasone in patients with proteasome inhibitor exposed and lenalidomide-refractory myeloma (trial MM-005). Blood. 2015;126:3036.
73. Lacy MQ, LaPlant BR, Laumann KM, Kumar S, Gertz MA, Hayman SR, Buadi F, Dispenzieri A, Lust JA, Kapoor P, et al. Pomalidomide, bortezomib and dexamethasone (PVD) for patients with relapsed lenalidomide refractory multiple myeloma (MM). Blood. 2014;124:304.
74. Voorhees PM, Mulkey F, Hassoun H, Paba-Prada CE, Efebera YA, Hoke E, Aquino G, Carlisle D, Suman V, Richardson PG. Alliance A061202. A phase I/II study of pomalidomide, dexamethasone and ixazomib versus pomalidomide and dexamethasone for patients

with multiple myeloma refractory to lenalidomide and proteasome inhibitor based therapy: phase I results. Blood. 2015;126:375.

75. Hsi ED, Steinle R, Balasa B, Szmania S, Draksharapu A, Shum BP, Huseni M, Powers D, Nanisetti A, Zhang Y, et al. CS1, a potential new therapeutic antibody target for the treatment of multiple myeloma. Clin Cancer Res. 2008;14:2775–84.

76. Tai YT, Dillon M, Song W, Leiba M, Li XF, Burger P, Lee AI, Podar K, Hideshima T, Rice AG, et al. Anti-CS1 humanized monoclonal antibody HuLuc63 inhibits myeloma cell adhesion and induces antibody-dependent cellular cytotoxicity in the bone marrow milieu. Blood. 2008;112:1329–37.

77. Collins SM, Bakan CE, Swartzel GD, Hofmeister CC, Efebera YA, Kwon H, Starling GC, Ciarlariello D, Bhaskar S, Briercheck EL, et al. Elotuzumab directly enhances NK cell cytotoxicity against myeloma via CS1 ligation: evidence for augmented NK cell function complementing ADCC. Cancer Immunol Immunother. 2013;62:1841–9.

78. Zonder JA, Mohrbacher AF, Singhal S, van Rhee F, Bensinger WI, Ding H, Fry J, Afar DE, Singhal AK. A phase 1, multicenter, open-label, dose escalation study of elotuzumab in patients with advanced multiple myeloma. Blood. 2012;120:552–9.

79. Richardson PG, Jagannath S, Moreau P, Jakubowiak A, Raab MS, Facon T, Vij R, White D, Reece DE, Benboubker L, et al. Final results for the 1703 phase 1b/2 study of elotuzumab in combination with lenalidomide and dexamethasone in patients with relapsed/refractory multiple myeloma. Blood. 2014b;124:302.

80. Lin P, Owens R, Tricot G, Wilson CS. Flow cytometric immunophenotypic analysis of 306 cases of multiple myeloma. Am J Clin Pathol. 2004;121:482–8.

81. Lokhorst HM, Plesner T, Laubach JP, Nahi H, Gimsing P, Hansson M, Minnema MC, Lassen U, Krejcik J, Palumbo A, et al. Targeting CD38 with Daratumumab Monotherapy in multiple myeloma. N Engl J Med. 2015;373:1207–19.

82. Lonial S, Weiss BM, Usmani SZ, Singhal S, Chari A, Bahlis NJ, Belch A, Krishnan A, Vescio RA, Mateos MV, et al. Daratumumab monotherapy in patients with treatment-refractory multiple myeloma (SIRIUS): an open-label, randomised, phase 2 trial. Lancet. 2016;387(10027):1551–60.

83. Dimopoulos MA, Oriol A, Nahi H, San Miguel J, Bahlis NJ, Rabin N, Orlowski R, Komarnicki M, Suzuki K, Plesner T, et al. An open-label, randomised phase 3 study of daratumumab, lenalidomide, and dexamethasone (DRd) versus lenalidomide and dexamethasone (Rd) in relapsed or refractory multiple myeloma (RRMM): POLLUX. European Hematology Association, Abstract LB2238; 2016b.

84. Kumar S, Flinn I, Richardson PG, Hari P, Callander N, Noga SJ, Stewart AK, Turturro F, Rifkin R, Wolf J, et al. Randomized, multicenter, phase 2 study (EVOLUTION) of combinations of bortezomib, dexamethasone, cyclophosphamide, and lenalidomide in previously untreated multiple myeloma. Blood. 2012;119:4375–82.

85. Monge J, Kortüm KM, Stewart AK, Bergsagel PL, Mikhael J, Reeder CB, Mayo A, Fonseca R. Cyclophosphamide, bortezomib, and dexamethasone (CYBORD) treatment for relapsed/refractory multiple myeloma. J Clin Oncol. 2014;32(suppl):8586.

86. Bringhen S, Petrucci MT, Larocca A, Conticello C, Rossi D, Magarotto V, Musto P, Boccadifuoco L, Offidani M, Omede P, et al. Carfilzomib, cyclophosphamide, and dexamethasone in patients with newly diagnosed multiple myeloma: a multicenter, phase 2 study. Blood. 2014;124:63–9.

87. Yong KL, Brown S, Hinsley S, Flanagan L, Rabin N, Ramasamy K, Cavenagh J, Owen RG, Kaiser MF, Low E, et al. Carfilzomib, cyclophosphamide and dexamethasone is well tolerated in patients with relapsed/refractory multiple myeloma who have received one prior regimen. Blood. 2015;126:1840.

88. Griffin PT, Ho VQ, Fulp W, Nishihori T, Shain KH, Alsina M, Baz RC. A comparison of salvage infusional chemotherapy regimens for recurrent/refractory multiple myeloma. Cancer. 2015;121:3622–30.

89. Holstein SA, Richardson PG, Laubach JP, McCarthy PL. Management of relapsed multiple myeloma after autologous stem cell transplant. Biol Blood Marrow Transplant. 2015;21: 793–8.

90. Jimenez-Zepeda VH, Mikhael J, Winter A, Franke N, Masih-Khan E, Trudel S, Chen C, Kukreti V, Reece DE. Second autologous stem cell transplantation as salvage therapy for multiple myeloma: impact on progression-free and overall survival. Biol Blood Marrow Transplant. 2012;18:773–9.

91. Michaelis LC, Saad A, Zhong X, Le-Rademacher J, Freytes CO, Marks DI, Lazarus HM, Bird JM, Holmberg L, Kamble RT, et al. Salvage second hematopoietic cell transplantation in myeloma. Biol Blood Marrow Transplant. 2013;19:760–6.

92. Chow AW, Lee CH, Hiwase DK, To LB, Horvath N. Relapsed multiple myeloma: who benefits from salvage autografts? Intern Med J. 2013;43:156–61.

93. Alvares CL, Davies FE, Horton C, Patel G, Powles R, Morgan GJ. The role of second autografts in the management of myeloma at first relapse. Haematologica. 2006;91:141–2.

94. Cook G, Williams C, Brown JM, Cairns DA, Cavenagh J, Snowden JA, Ashcroft AJ, Fletcher M, Parrish C, Yong K, et al. High-dose chemotherapy plus autologous stem-cell transplantation as consolidation therapy in patients with relapsed multiple myeloma after previous autologous stem-cell transplantation (NCRI myeloma X relapse [intensive trial]): a randomised, open-label, phase 3 trial. Lancet Oncol. 2014;15:874–85.

95. Cook G, Williams C, Cairns DA, Hockaday A, Cavenagh J, Snowden JA, Parrish C, Yong KL, Cavet J, Hunter H, et al. A salvage autologous stem cell transplant (ASCT2) induces superior overall survival following bortezomib-containing re-induction therapy for relapsed multiple myeloma (MM): results from the myeloma X (intensive) trial. Blood. 2015;126:394.

96. Freytes CO, Vesole DH, LeRademacher J, Zhong X, Gale RP, Kyle RA, Reece DE, Gibson J, Schouten HC, McCarthy PL, et al. Second transplants for multiple myeloma relapsing after a previous autotransplant-reduced-intensity allogeneic vs autologous transplantation. Bone Marrow Transplant. 2014;49:416–21.

97. Kumar S, Mahmood ST, Lacy MQ, Dispenzieri A, Hayman SR, Buadi FK, Dingli D, Rajkumar SV, Litzow MR, Gertz MA. Impact of early relapse after auto-SCT for multiple myeloma. Bone Marrow Transplant. 2008a;42:413–20.

98. Jimenez-Zepeda VH, Reece DE, Trudel S, Chen C, Tiedemann R, Kukreti V. Early relapse after single auto-SCT for multiple myeloma is a major predictor of survival in the era of novel agents. Bone Marrow Transplant. 2015;50:204–8.

99. Kuczynski EA, Sargent DJ, Grothey A, Kerbel RS. Drug rechallenge and treatment beyond progression--implications for drug resistance. Nat Rev Clin Oncol. 2013;10:571–87.

100. Petrucci MT, Giraldo P, Corradini P, Teixeira A, Dimopoulos MA, Blau IW, Drach J, Angermund R, Allietta N, Broer E, et al. A prospective, international phase 2 study of bortezomib retreatment in patients with relapsed multiple myeloma. Br J Haematol. 2013;160:649–59.

101. Mateos MV, Richardson PG, Schlag R, Khuageva NK, Dimopoulos MA, Shpilberg O, Kropff M, Spicka I, Petrucci MT, Palumbo A, et al. Bortezomib plus melphalan and prednisone compared with melphalan and prednisone in previously untreated multiple myeloma: updated follow-up and impact of subsequent therapy in the phase III VISTA trial. J Clin Oncol. 2010;28:2259–66.

102. Madan S, Lacy MQ, Dispenzieri A, Gertz MA, Buadi F, Hayman SR, Detweiler-Short K, Dingli D, Zeldenrust S, Lust J, et al. Efficacy of retreatment with immunomodulatory drugs (IMiDs) in patients receiving IMiDs for initial therapy of newly diagnosed multiple myeloma. Blood. 2011;118:1763–5.

Treatment of Patients in Third Relapse and Beyond Including Double-Refractory Disease

Douglas Tremblay, Siyang Leng, and Ajai Chari

6.1 Introduction

In the last 15 years, the approval of multiple new anti-myeloma agents has led to significant improvement in outcomes for patients with relapsed and refractory disease. However, the expanded repertoire of treatment options produces increasingly complex treatment decisions. Patients experiencing a third relapse or beyond typically have more aggressive disease and are heavily pretreated, making their treatment choices more challenging. This is highlighted in a prospective database of 578 patients, where the median event-free survival for the third, fourth, and fifth relapse were 6, 4.5, and 4 months, respectively. This is in contrast to event-free survival of first and second relapses that were 10 and 7 months, respectively, highlighting that a remission after third relapses is generally less durable [1]. Even in the era of novel therapies, patients refractory to treatment have poor outcomes.

In addition to the number of relapses, double-refractory disease (i.e., refractory to both bortezomib and thalidomide or lenalidomide), in particular, carries an extremely poor prognosis, with a progression-free survival (PFS) of 5 months and overall survival (OS) of 9 months [2]. There are many options from currently available classes of therapies (Table 6.1). In the setting of double-refractory disease, second-generation proteasome inhibitor carfilzomib and third-generation immunomodulatory (IMiD) pomalidomide have demonstrated efficacy. These and the other approved agents have been explored in combination therapy (Table 6.2). The histone deacetylase inhibitor (HDAC) inhibitors (e.g. panobinostat) are promising agents, particularly in combination therapy. Unfortunately, the survival of patients with multiple relapses and double-refractory disease remains poor, highlighting the

D. Tremblay, M.D. • S. Leng, M.D. • A. Chari, M.D. (✉)
Multiple Myeloma Program, Icahn School of Medicine at Mount Sinai,
One Gustave L. Levy Place, Box 1185, New York, NY 10029-6574, USA
e-mail: ajai.chari@mssm.edu

© Springer International Publishing AG 2018
S.Z. Usmani, A.K. Nooka (eds.), *Personalized Therapy for Multiple Myeloma*,
https://doi.org/10.1007/978-3-319-61872-2_6

Table 6.1 Currently available therapies

Steroids	IMiDs	Proteasome inhibitors	Conventional chemotherapy	HDAC inhibitors	Monoclonal antibodies
Prednisone	Thalidomide	Bortezomib	Melphalan	Panobinostat	Daratumumab
Dexamethasone	Lenalidomide	Carfilzomib	Cyclophosphamide		Elotuzumab
	Pomalidomide	Ixazomib	Liposomal doxorubicin		
			DCEP/D-PACE		
			Carmustine (BCNU)		
			Bendamustine		

DCEP Dexamethasone, cyclophosphamide, etoposide, cisplatin; *D-PACE* Dexamethasone, cisplatin, doxorubicin, cyclophosphamide, etoposide; *HDAC* histone deacetylase; *IMiDs* immunomodulators

Table 6.2 Efficacy of combination therapy in relapsed/refractory multiple myeloma

	Phase	n	IMiD exposed	PI exposed (%)	ORR (%)	PFS (months)	OS (months)	Reference
Doublet therapy								
Thalidomide	2	169	0%	0	30	2 years: 20%	2 years: 48%	[3]
Bort + Dex	3	669	49%	0	38	6.22	30	[4]
Bort + Doxil vs. Bort	3	646	41%	0	43	9	33	[5]
Len Dex MM009	3	177	41%	10	61	11.1	29.6	[6]
Len Dex MM010	3	349	30%	4.50	60	11.3	38	[7]
Car (+Dex 8)	2	266	100%	9	23.7	3.7	15.6	[8]
Pom Dex vs. Dex	3	302	100%	95	31	4.2	13.1	[9]
Triplet therapy								
Bort Thal Dex	1–2	85	74%	0	65	6	22	[10]
Bort Len Dex	2	64	73%T, 6%L	53	64	9.5	30	[11]
Bort Pom Dex	1	28	100%	100	71	NA	NA	[12]
Car Len Dex	2	52	73%	80	77	15.4	NA	[13]
Car Pom Dex	1–2	79	100%	97	50	7.2	20.6	[14]

Bort bortezomib, *Car* carfilzomib, *Dex* dexamethasone, *Len* lenalidomide, *Pom* pomalidomide

need for a better understanding of the biology of multiple myeloma to develop novel agents and targeted therapies.

This chapter will review the currently available therapies for patients experiencing third relapse after at least two lines of therapy, as well as the treatment of double-refractory disease, with a particular attention paid toward novel therapies in development for aggressive, relapsing myeloma.

6.2 Factors Affecting Selection of Therapy

6.2.1 Biochemical Versus Symptomatic Relapse

Patients who present with a biochemical relapse but without worsening in symptoms may, under certain circumstances, be observed before initiating salvage therapy. However, even in the absence of symptoms, if there is a history of complications from myeloma, known high-risk disease, or high tumor burden, treatment should likely be initiated sooner rather than later.

6.2.2 Patient Comorbidities

Patients may suffer from renal impairment, hepatic impairment, and other comorbidities which may affect the selection of an agent at relapse. Renal impairment, from disease related or other comorbidities, should not affect the dose of corticosteroids, proteasome inhibitors [15], thalidomide [16], pomalidomide [17, 18], cyclophosphamide [19], liposomal doxorubicin [20], bendamustine [21], and panobinostat [22]. However, treatment with lenalidomide and melphalan requires dose adjustment, as decreased renal clearance causes increases in blood levels and resultant worsening myelosuppression [23]. Additionally, personalized strategies for elderly patients, with particular attention being paid to the assessment of their frailty, comorbidities, and disabilities, would likely improve tolerability and outcomes [24].

6.2.3 Prior Drug Exposures

Reviewing prior drug exposures is crucial to determining a treatment plan for relapsed or refractory disease. Patients who have not been exposed to particular IMiDs or PIs, for example, should be treated with regimens containing these. Even if patients have been exposed to particular agent, if a drug was well tolerated and produced a response that was durable, without relapse for over 6 months, they may benefit from re-treatment. While many agents (e.g., lenalidomide, pomalidomide, carfilzomib) are used until progression, initial bortezomib studies were given for fixed duration. In the RETRIEVE trial, 130 relapsed patients who had previously responded to bortezomib were retreated with bortezomib plus dexamethasone. The overall response rate (ORR) was 40%, without a cumulative toxicity burden [25].

A meta-analysis including 1051 patients who were relapsed or refractory retreated with bortezomib showed that ORR was 39.1%. Relapsed patients had a higher ORR than refractory patients [26]. Taken together, these data suggest that bortezomib is efficacious in re-treatment, although this option is better reserved for relapsed rather than refractory patients.

6.2.4 Genomics

Cytogenetic abnormalities that portend a poorer prognosis may also dictate treatment. For instance, t(4;14) mutation is associated with worse event-free survival and overall survival [27]. However, bortezomib and carfilzomib treatment have been shown to improve EFS and OS in patients with t(4;14), thereby overcoming this mutation's negative prognostic value and resulting in reclassification as standard risk [28, 29].

Del(17p) is also associated with worse outcomes in patients with multiple myeloma [27]. Recently pomalidomide has demonstrated activity in patients with this cytogenetic abnormality, with improved 4-month PFS [30]. Additionally, ixazomib has also been shown to have a potentially favorable impact on the adverse prognosis conferred by high-risk genetic alterations. In combination with lenalidomide and dexamethasone, ixazomib increased PFS, with similar benefits seen in the del(17p) and t(4;14) subgroup [31]. Although these findings are promising, more research is required to understand the difference in cytogenetics at relapse and how it relates to prognosis and treatment decisions. Moreover, without phase III studies comparing novel therapy to conventional therapy stratified by standard-risk and high-risk disease, it is difficult to determine whether a novel agent merely improves the outcomes of high-risk feature or actually is able to overcome such risk [32].

Other genomic findings play a role in treatment as drugs typically reserved for treatment of other malignancies can be repurposed against myeloma in specific circumstances. For instance, patients with BRAF-mutated multiple myeloma may benefit from BRAF inhibitors. For instance, the BRAF inhibitor vemurafenib has been successfully used in two patients with BRAF-V600E-mutated MM [33]. MEK inhibitors are also actively being investigated given the implication of Ras/MAPK pathway in the pathogenesis MM [34]. These examples highlight how comprehensive genomic profiling can identify genomic driver mutations to develop a rationalized therapy plan. Commercially available assays have been utilized for this effect. For instance, 214 patients with multiple myeloma underwent comprehensive genomic profiling on CD138-selected bone marrow cells, showing 147 clinically relevant alterations [35].

6.3 Currently Available Drug Classes

6.3.1 Carfilzomib

Carfilzomib has demonstrated clinical benefit in relapsed myeloma with low number of prior lines of therapy in the ASPIRE trial [36] and when compared with bortezomib in the ENDEAVOR trial [37]. Carfilzomib is currently FDA approved at the dose of 27 mg/m^2 for the treatment of patients who have received at least two prior lines of therapy. However, at a higher dose of 56 mg/m^2, carfilzomib can safely be administered with an improved ORR of 55–77% [37, 38]. For patients who have progressed with standard dosing carfilzomib, they may be able to be recaptured with high dose. This has been demonstrated in our study of 13 patients refractory to carfilzomib 27 mg/m^2 with 4.5 median lines of prior therapy, who were given 56 mg/m^2 and had an ORR of 42%, with a clinical benefit rate (CBR, i.e., ≥ minor response) of 58% [39], with a larger, confirmatory randomized study led by SWOG.

6.3.2 Ixazomib

Ixazomib is an oral proteasome inhibitor. In phase I study, it was shown to have ORR of 15–20% and SD of 30–60% in the relapsed/refractory population [40, 41]. In the phase III tourmaline-MM1 study, patients with relapsed/refractory myeloma who were not refractory to lenalidomide or proteasome inhibitors were treated with ixazomib, lenalidomide, and dexamethasone. Compared to those who received lenalidomide and dexamethasone, the ixazomib had a significant PFS advantage at interim analysis—20.6 vs. 14.7 months, without a significant increase in toxicity [31]. On the basis of these results, ixazomib was recently approved in combination with lenalidomide and dexamethasone by the FDA for the treatment of myeloma in patients who have received at least one prior therapy.

Ixazomib has also been investigated in a phase I/II study in patients with double-refractory disease who were treated with ixazomib, pomalidomide, and dexamethasone. This regimen demonstrated a favorable side effect profile and a best ORR of 62% [42]. A phase I study of ixazomib and panobinostat is also under way in patients (10 out of 11 patients with double refractory), preliminary data showing that this regimen is well tolerated and has demonstrated three MRs [43]. Additional data about the efficacy of ixazomib in patients refractory to proteasome inhibitors is awaited, and numerous combination trials in refractory disease are under way.

6.3.3 Panobinostat

Panobinostat has demonstrated effectiveness in relapsed disease. In the phase III PANORAMA study, patients with 1–3 relapses were randomized to bortezomib with placebo or panobinostat. The panobinostat group had a PFS increase of 3.9 months compared to placebo [44]. More importantly for the multiply relapsed and refractory population, in the phase II PANORAMA 2 study, 55 heavily pre-treated bortezomib refractory patients were treated with panobinostat, bortezomib, and dexamethasone. The ORR was 34.5%; PFS was 5.4 months [45]. Panobinostat can also be used in combination with lenalidomide, as demonstrated in an ongoing phase II study, demonstrating an ORR of 41% with a CBR of 74%, including the activity in lenalidomide refractory patients ($N = 22$), with a 36% ORR and a median

PFS of 6.5 months [46]. Additionally, panobinostat in combination with carfilzomib has been explored as a therapeutic option in a phase I trial of patients with multiple relapses. An ORR of 50% was observed with 30% PR and 20% VGPR [47].

6.3.4 Pomalidomide

Pomalidomide, a thalidomide analog, has demonstrated anti-myeloma activity in vitro and has produced promising results for relapsed MM. In an open-label, international study of 455 patients with a median of 5 lines of prior therapy, patients were randomized to pomalidomide and dexamethasone versus high-dose dexamethasone alone. The trial was stopped early due to an interim analysis demonstrating a survival benefit for pomalidomide. In the pomalidomide group, PFS and OS were 3.8 months and 11.9 months, respectively. This is in contrast to the dexamethasone alone group, which had a PFS of 1.9 months and OS of 7.8 months. The ORR was 31% vs. 10% in favor of the pomalidomide group. This benefits to the overall survival and progression-free survival maintained in a subgroup analysis when including patients with more than two previous treatments, demonstrating effectiveness in third relapse and beyond [9].

Pomalidomide has also been used in combination therapy. In a phase I/II trial of pomalidomide, cyclophosphamide and prednisone, 55 patients received treatment with an ORR of 51% and a median PFS of 10.4 months [48]. Clarithromycin has been shown to improve the efficacy of lenalidomide, so it has also been explored in combination with pomalidomide. In a phase II trial, this combination produced an ORR of 56%, 23% greater than VGPR, and a median PFS of 5 months [49]. Finally, pomalidomide has been investigated in combination with carfilzomib. In a heavily pretreated population (median of 6 prior lines of therapy), this combination had an ORR of 50%, with a median PFS of 7.2 months [14].

6.3.5 Salvage ASCT

Patients who have undergone an ASCT as an initial therapy or during a prior relapse may benefit from a second ASCT. A retrospective study at the Mayo Clinic of 98 patients who underwent salvage ASCT, with a median of 3 prior chemotherapeutic agents, showed a PFS of 10.3 months with a median OS from the second ASCT of 33 months. Higher number of treatment regimens prior to salvage ASCT predicted shorter PFS; however, OS was only shorter in patients who had a shorter time to progression after their first ASCT. Therefore, salvage ASCT should be considered as a therapeutic option during third relapse and beyond, particularly if a PFS was longer than 12 months after the first ASCT, or alternatively, to improve hematopoietic reserve in those patients with heavy marrow replacement, as a bridge to subsequent therapy [50].

6.4   Novel Drug Classes

Despite the approval of carfilzomib, pomalidomide, and panobinostat, there is a continued need for newer agents as patients continue to have remissions. While many agents demonstrate preclinical anti-myeloma activity, few demonstrate clinically meaningful activity. A recent retrospective review of over 129 drugs explored as single agents in clinical trials demonstrated that only drugs with a mean response rate of 15% are in current clinical use. Additionally, all currently commonly used therapies had a RR of at least 20% [51]. This provides a framework for prioritizing large-scale phase III trials. Therefore, this section will only focus on agents (Table 6.3) that have achieved a single-agent response rate of at least 15–20% or, alternatively, have overcome drug resistance, as these are the agents most likely to be clinically relevant in the future.

6.4.1   Proteasome Inhibitor

Given the success of bortezomib and carfilzomib, there is now an active interest in the development of novel PIs for the treatment of relapsed MM. Marizomib is a marine-derived irreversible proteasome inhibitor which inhibits all three protease activities—chymotrypsin-like, trypsin-like, and caspase-like—of the 20S proteasome in a manner distinct from that of bortezomib or carfilzomib. Preclinical studies suggest that cross-resistance to marizomib does not occur after exposure to other proteasome inhibitors [52]. A phase I/II clinical trial of marizomib with or without dexamethasone is ongoing. Thirty-four patients with relapsed/refractory MM (median 6 prior regimens) have been treated. Of 15 patients who had received the therapeutic dose range, three (all bortezomib refractory) attained PR (20%). Dose-limiting toxicities included transient hallucinations, cognitive changes, and loss of balance, all of which were reversible and consistent with the drug's ability to penetrate the blood-brain barrier [53]. In a phase I study examining marizomib in combination with pomalidomide and low-dose dexamethasone in a population with a median of 5 prior lines of therapy, the ORR was 64% ($n = 17$). Grade 3/4 AEs included neutropenia (32%), anemia (9%), thrombocytopenia (9%), and pneumonia (9%) [54].

Table 6.3 Novel therapeutic classes

Cell cycle/apoptosis	Kinase inhibitors	Monoclonal antibodies	Immune modulators
Filanesib	Dinaciclib	Daratumumab	Pembrolizumab
Selinexor	Afuseritib	Isatuximab	CAR-T cells
	LGH447	Indatuximab ravtansine	

6.4.2 HDAC6 Inhibitor

Ricolinostat is an oral selective HDAC6 inhibitor which has shown promising pre-clinical synergy with lenalidomide and pomalidomide [55]. Although tolerated as a monotherapy, it is currently being evaluated in the context of combination therapy. In an ongoing phase I/II of patients (median 4 lines of prior therapy), combination ricolinostat, pomalidomide, and dexamethasone demonstrated an ORR of 29%, including three VGPR. Common toxicities include fatigue, diarrhea, and cytopenias [56]. Additionally, ricolinostat has been combined with bortezomib and dexamethasone that produced an ORR of 32% in 48 heavily pretreated patients (5 median lines of therapy) [57]. Taken together, these data are promising for ricolinostat as a clinically efficacious agent in relapsed and refractory myeloma.

6.4.3 Cell Cycle Inhibitor

Filanesib is a kinesin spindle protein inhibitor. Kinesin spindle proteins play an integral role in mitosis by mediating centrosome separation and assembly of the bipolar spindle. By blocking these proteins, filanesib results in a monopolar spindle thereby leading to mitotic arrest and apoptosis [58]. A phase I study examined the single-agent safety, pharmacokinetics, and activity of filanesib in patients with relapsed or refractory myeloma. Thirty-one patients were reported, with a median of six prior regimens, and all had received a proteasome inhibitor (PI) and an IMiD in the past. Among the 31 evaluable patients, there were three confirmed PRs and one confirmed MR. The most common AEs were hematologic [59]. It was subsequently found that filanesib can be bound by the acute-phase reactant protein α-1 acid glycoprotein (AAG), and higher levels of AAG result in inferior outcomes with filanesib therapy. In patients with low AAG levels, the single-agent response rate was 24% [60].

A phase I study is examining the combination of bortezomib and filanesib. Recruited patients had relapsed/refractory disease with a median of 5 prior lines of therapy. Among 13 evaluable patients, 4 PR (31%) and 1 minor response (MR) were observed [61]. A phase II study is examining the combination of carfilzomib with or without filanesib. Of 50 evaluable patients (randomized in a 2:1 fashion), the ORR was 10% in the carfilzomib arm and 30% in the carfilzomib + filanesib arm. Grade 3/4 AEs in proteasome inhibitor and filanesib combination studies are predominantly hematologic [62].

6.4.4 Apoptosis Inducer

Selinexor (KPT-330) is an oral selective inhibitor of the nuclear export protein CRM1/XPO1. The chromosome region maintenance 1 (CRM1) is highly expressed in MM, particularly in cells resistant to bortezomib. Selinexor induces the accumulation of CRM1 protein with MM cells as well as the retention of multiple tumor suppressor proteins such as p53, pRB, CDKN2A, p21, and FOXO, leading to growth arrest and apoptosis. It has also been shown to block NF-kB and resensitize cells to bortezomib [63]. An ongoing phase I open-label dose-escalation study is examining the use of selinexor in patients with hematologic malignancies. Among 40 evaluable MM patients, in the >65 mg (approximately 35 mg/m^2) group, there was 1 CR (3%), 6 PRs (21%), and 6 MRs (21%), giving an ORR of 24%. Grade 3/4 toxicities were predominantly hematologic with non-hematologic toxicities such as nausea, anorexia, and hypokalemia being all <5% [64]. The addition of dexamethasone to selinexor was investigated in a phase I study of 28 patients with refractory MM with a median of 6 prior regimens (including pomalidomide (68%) and carfilzomib (36%)) who were given selinexor at 30–60 mg/m^2 with either 0, <20, or 20 mg dexamethasone. For the selinexor 45 mg/m^2 and dexamethasone 20 mg doses, ORR was 60%, with 1 attaining sCR (10%) and 5 PR (50%). The reported AEs were Grade 1–2 and were nausea, fatigue, anorexia, and vomiting [65].

Another ongoing phase I study is examining selinexor in combination with carfilzomib. Of eight enrolled patients, all had relapsed/refractory MM with a median of five prior treatment regimens. Six were refractory to carfilzomib combinations. No DLTs have yet been noted, and the MTD has not been established. For response, 1 has attained VGPR (12.5%) and 6 PR (75%). Responses occurred rapidly (typically 1 cycle), although some patients also progressed fairly quickly (after 1, 2, 4, and 4 months). Grade 3–4 AEs were hematologic and also fatigue (25%) and upper respiratory tract infection (25%) [66].

6.4.5   Protein Kinase Inhibitors

Despite the approval signal transduction inhibitors in other B-cell malignancies, to date there is no such agent approved for myeloma. Ibrutinib, an oral covalent inhibitor of Bruton's tyrosine kinase (BTK), is FDA approved for the treatment of previously treated chronic lymphocytic leukemia, mantle cell lymphoma, and Waldenström's macroglobulinemia. As a single agent in patients with myeloma, it has shown clinical benefit to previously treated disease demonstrating a CBR of 23%, with sustained SR (greater than 4 cycles) in 30% [67]. Recently, ibrutinib has also been investigated in combination with carfilzomib in the relapsed and refractory setting. In a phase I trial of 40 patients, an ORR of 62% was achieved, including an ORR of 62% in patients refractory to bortezomib. The treatment was well tolerated, with the most common adverse effects being hypertension, anemia, pneumonia, and thrombocytopenia [68].

Cyclin-dependent kinases regulate progression through the cell cycle and can be dysregulated by immunoglobulin (Ig)H translocations, which is common in MM. Dinaciclib is a small molecular inhibitor of CDKs. It has been investigated as a single agent in a phase I/II trial of 27 patients with recurrent MM but with less than 5 lines of therapy. Two patients achieved a VGPR, and 10 patients achieved M-protein stabilization [69].

Afuresertib is an oral, reversible, pan-AKT kinase inhibitor. AKT is a serine/threonine kinase that is a key mediator of PI3K-mTOR signaling, a pathway which has been found to be upregulated in many cancers including MM. A phase I study examined the use of afuresertib in 73 patients, 34 of whom had MM. Among the myeloma cohort, median line of prior therapies was 5.5. Three patients (9%) attained PRs, and three more attained MRs. The most frequent AEs were nausea (36%), diarrhea (33%), and dyspepsia (25%) [70]. A phase Ib/II study examined the use of afuresertib in combination with bortezomib and dexamethasone. Sixty-seven patients with relapsed MM were reported, with a median of 3.5 prior lines of therapy. ORR was 61%, with 1 CR, 3 VGPR, 10 PR, and 3 MR noted. Grade 3/4 AEs were thrombocytopenia (28%), diarrhea 913%), rash (13%), and anemia (10%) [71].

LGH447 is a novel, pan-Pim kinase inhibitor that has been investigated in patients with relapsed myeloma. In a phase I trial of heavily pretreated patients, an RR of 10.5% was observed [72]. While the single-agent activity of these protein kinase inhibitors does not meet the 20% RR required for investment of further investigation, these agents may be useful in combination with other agents.

6.5   Immunologic Approaches

6.5.1   Monoclonal Antibodies

A promising therapeutic strategy is targeting antigens expressed on myeloma cells with monoclonal antibodies, therapy inducing apoptosis, or growth arrest. Daratumumab is a novel monoclonal antibody against CD38, a transmembrane glycoprotein expressed in the majority of myeloma cells. In one phase I–II clinical trial of heavily pretreated patients, 42% had a PR with doses of >4 mg/kg [73]. In an ongoing phase II study, 106 patients with a median of 5 lines or prior therapy administered daratumumab at 16 mg/kg showed an ORR of 29.2%, including three patients who experienced a sCR. The median duration of response was 7.4 months. The most common side effects were fatigue, cytopenias, and cough [74]. Infusion reactions occurred in 43% of patients, predominantly grade 1 and 2 with only 5% grade 3 and no grade 4 reactions. More than 90% of infusion reactions occurred during the first infusion and were much less common in subsequent infusions. Since CD38 is also expressed on red blood cells, daratumumab can also result in a universally positive indirect antibody (or indirect Coombs) test, so red blood cell typing should be performed immediately prior to daratumumab administration to establish a true baseline [75]. On the basis of this phase II study, daratumumab was designated a "breakthrough therapy" by the FDA and on November 16, 2015, approved for subjects with greater than 3 lines of therapy or IMiD and PI refractory.

Daratumumab is also being explored as combination therapy. Lenalidomide plus daratumumab is being investigated in 32 patients with relapsed myeloma, demonstrating an ORR of 88%. Additionally, responses deepened over time in 61% of responders [76]. Daratumumab and pomalidomide are also being investigated. In an ongoing, multicenter phase Ib trial, in 98 patients, the ORR was 71%, including

67% in double-refractory patients. Additionally, there was no added toxicity aside from daratumumab-related infusion reactions [77].

Elotuzumab is an immunostimulatory monoclonal antibody which targets signaling lymphocytic activation molecule F7 (SLAMF7), which is highly expressed on myeloma cells. It has demonstrated clinical efficacy in combination with lenalidomide and dexamethasone in patients with 1–3 prior lines of therapy [78]. It has also been investigated in combination with bortezomib and dexamethasone. One hundred and fifty-two patients with 1–3 prior lines of therapy were randomized to elotuzumab, bortezomib, dexamethasone or bortezomib, and dexamethasone alone. 51% in the treatment arm and 53% in the control arm had prior PI exposure. After a median number of 12 treatment cycles, PFS was 9.9 months in the elotuzumab group and 6.8 months in the control arm [79]. A study of elotuzumab in combination with pomalidomide and dexamethasone is also nearly open to accrual.

Isatuximab (SAR650984) is a humanized monoclonal antibody that selectively binds selectively to human CD38 receptor. It exerts anti-myeloma affect via ADCC, CDC, and direct apoptosis. In a phase II trial in patients with heavily pretreated myeloma, an ORR of 24–29% was observed. Fatigue and anemia were the most common treatment-emergent adverse events [80].

Indatuximab ravtansine is an antibody-drug conjugate comprised of anti-CD138 chimerized monoclonal antibody and the maytansinoid DM4. It binds to CD138 on cancer cells and releases DM4 to induce cell death. Although it is not efficacious as a single agent, it has shown promising results in combination therapy with lenalidomide. In a phase I/IIa trial of patients refractory to lenalidomide, the combination of indatuximab ravtansine and lenalidomide produced a 78% ORR and 100% clinical benefit, including 73% in lenalidomide refractory patients [81]. With greater understanding of the biology of MM, monoclonal antibodies are likely to play a major role in treating patients with multiple relapses.

6.5.2   Tumor Vaccination and Oncolytic Viruses

Another future direction in relapsed and refractory disease is utilizing the immune system to produce a myeloma-specific response to eliminate residual disease. Dendritic cell-based tumor vaccines are a promising means to selectively eliminate malignant cells. This has been explored in a phase I trial of 17 generally heavily pretreated patients (mean 4 prior treatments). These patients underwent serial vaccination with the dendritic cell/multiple myeloma fusions in conjunction with granulocyte macrophage colony-stimulating factor. There was a tenfold expansion in myeloma-reactive T cells and disease stabilization in 66% of patients [82]. This strategy has also been explored in conjunction with ASCT in less treatment-experienced patients [83]. Using immune modulators such as lenalidomide has preclinical evidence of enhancing response to dendritic cell/multiple myeloma fusions [84] and is being investigated in ongoing clinical trials as maintenance after ASCT.

6.5.3   Allogeneic Stem Cell Transplant

Allogeneic stem cell transplant (allo-SCT) may represent the only potentially cura-tive option for patients with MM. Unfortunately, due to high treatment-related mor-tality, the appropriate patient population for this therapy is restricted. Additionally, treatment with novel agents in conjunction with ASCT is improving survival, mak-ing the role of allo-SCT unclear. Myeloablative allo-SCT has fallen out of favor given the high treatment-related mortality. For instance, one study of 80 highly treatment-experienced patients undergoing myeloablative allo-ASCT showed 44% died of treatment-related complications [85]. In an attempt to mitigate these compli-cations, nonmyeloablative allo-SCT has been further investigated in relapsed myeloma.

Allo-SCT after ASCT has been explored in a phase III study, without a clear benefit of incorporating an allo-SCT. Seven hundred and ten patients who had received ASCT were randomized to allo-SCT (auto-allo) or another ASCT (auto-auto). Three-year Kaplan-Meier estimates of PFS were 43% in the auto-allo and 46% in the auto-auto; OS did not differ between the two groups. Adverse events also did not significantly differ between the two groups [76].

T-cell-depleted allo-SCT attempts to decrease the rates of graft-versus-host dis-ease (GVHD) and represents an emerging potential therapy for high-risk refractory myeloma. In a phase II clinical trial, the percentage of patient with PFS and OS at 2 years were 31% and 54%, respectively. Additionally, there were only 2% of patients who had acute GVHD, and none had chronic GVHD. Transplant-related mortality was 18% [86]. Further prospective trials are needed to evaluate the effi-cacy of this intervention in the relapsed setting.

6.5.4   Immune Modulators

Given the unclear role of allogeneic transplantation in myeloma relative to other hematologic malignancies, there is a great deal of excitement regarding novel immune modulators in myeloma. The interaction of PD-L1, a transmembrane pro-tein expressed on MM cells, and PD-1 represents an attractive therapeutic target. Anti-PD-L1 and anti-PD-1 antibodies are available and have been preliminarily tested in advanced solid malignancies, showing a favorable safety profile and dura-ble response [87, 88]. Clinical trials using anti-PD-L1 antibodies as a single agent or in conjunction with lenalidomide are underway. Pembrolizumab, a highly selec-tive anti-PD-1 monoclonal antibody, has been tested in combination with lenalido-mide and dexamethasone in patients with refractory myeloma and resulted in an ORR of 76% ($n = 17$) and, interestingly, a 56% ORR in lenalidomide refractory patients (albeit $n = 9$) [89]. Pembrolizumab has also been investigated in combina-tion with pomalidomide and dexamethasone in an ongoing phase II study in 24 patients; 75% of which were double refractory to both PIs and IMiDs. An ORR of 50% was observed, including three patients with a near CR [90].

Chimeric antigen receptor (CAR) T cells provide another potentially promising therapeutic avenue. Engineering T cells to recognize specific myeloma cells, as demonstrated in other malignancies, may be possible. One case report demonstrated a sustained, complete response in a patient treated with CAR-T cells against CD19 in conjunction with standard myeloma therapies [82]. In an ongoing, recently reported first-in-humans clinical trial of CAR-T cell expressing anti-B-cell maturation antigen (BCMA), 11 patients with a median of 7 prior lines of therapy were given cyclophosphamide and fludarabine to deplete endogenous leukocytes and then received an infusion CAR-BCMA T cells at four dose levels. Of six patients treated with the lowest two dose levels, one patient experienced a PR, while the other five had SD. On the third dose level, two patients had SD, and one had a VGPR. Of the two patients who received the highest dose levels, one had a sCR, although both patients' courses were complicated by cytokine release syndrome [83]. These data, although preliminary, demonstrate promising anti-myeloma activity of anti-BCMA CAR-T cells and represent a promising line of potential therapy.

Conclusions

Multiply relapsed and refractory myeloma present many challenges. One can expect a more aggressive course than prior lines of therapy. Additionally, there are only limited, FDA-approved therapies available. A clinician designed a treatment strategy that must consider the nature of the patient's relapse, prior drug exposures, and comorbidities. Genomic data may also influence the decision, with attention to del(17p), which would favor choosing pomalidomide. Testing for specific mutations with therapeutic agents (e.g., BRAF) will likely become more prevalent as the treatment of myeloma becomes more personalized.

Despite the challenging aspect of myeloma that has multiple relapses, there are promising advances, such as the recent approval of daratumumab. With increased understanding of the biology driving myeloma, novel therapeutic agents are being developed and many have yielded promising phase I/II results. With this explosion in new agents, it will become even more important to prioritize therapies that have a high likelihood of success, with a RR of 15–20% or overcoming drug resistance. The development of these new therapies will continue to transform multiple myeloma from a terminal illness into a manageable, chronic disease.

References

1. Kumar SK, Therneau TM, Gertz MA, et al. Clinical course of patients with relapsed multiple myeloma. Mayo Clin Proc. 2004;79:867–74. doi:10.1016/S0025-6196(11)62152-6.
2. Kumar SK, Lee JH, Lahuerta JJ, et al. Risk of progression and survival in multiple myeloma relapsing after therapy with IMiDs and bortezomib: a multicenter international myeloma working group study. Leukemia. 2012;26:149–57. doi:10.1038/leu.2011.196.
3. Barlogie B, Desikan R, Eddlemon P, et al. Extended survival in advanced and refractory multiple myeloma after single-agent thalidomide: identification of prognostic factors in a phase 2 study of 169 patients. Blood. 2001;98:492–4.
4. Richardson PG, Sonneveld P, Schuster MW, et al. Bortezomib or high-dose dexamethasone for relapsed multiple myeloma. N Engl J Med. 2005;352:2487–98. doi:10.1056/NEJMoa043445.

5. Orlowski RZ, Nagler A, Sonneveld P, et al. Randomized phase III study of pegylated liposomal doxorubicin plus bortezomib compared with bortezomib alone in relapsed or refractory multiple myeloma: combination therapy improves time to progression. J Clin Oncol. 2007;25:3892–901. doi:10.1200/JCO.2006.10.5460.

6. Weber DM, Chen C, Niesvizky R, et al. Lenalidomide plus dexamethasone for relapsed multiple myeloma in North America. N Engl J Med. 2007;357:2133–42. doi:10.1056/NEJMoa070596.

7. Dimopoulos M, Spencer A, Attal M, et al. Lenalidomide plus dexamethasone for relapsed or refractory multiple myeloma. N Engl J Med. 2007;357:2123–32. doi:10.1056/NEJMoa070594.

8. Siegel DS, Martin T, Wang M, et al. A phase 2 study of single-agent carfilzomib (PX-171-003-A1) in patients with relapsed and refractory multiple myeloma. Blood. 2012;120:2817–25. doi:10.1182/blood-2012-05-425934.

9. San Miguel J, Weisel K, Moreau P, et al. Pomalidomide plus low-dose dexamethasone versus high-dose dexamethasone alone for patients with relapsed and refractory multiple myeloma (MM-003): a randomised, open-label, phase 3 trial. Lancet Oncol. 2013;14:1055–66. doi:10.1016/S1470-2045(13)70380-2.

10. Pineda-Roman M, Zangari M, van Rhee F, et al. VTD combination therapy with bortezomib-thalidomide-dexamethasone is highly effective in advanced and refractory multiple myeloma. Leukemia. 2008;22:1419–27. doi:10.1038/leu.2008.99.

11. Richardson PG, Xie W, Jagannath S, et al. A phase 2 trial of lenalidomide, bortezomib, and dexamethasone in patients with relapsed and relapsed/refractory myeloma. Blood. 2014;123:1461–9. doi:10.1182/blood-2013-07-517276.

12. Richardson PG, Hofmeister C, Raje NS, et al. MM-005: phase 1 trial of pomalidomide (POM), bortezomib (BORT), and low-dose dexamethasone (LoDEX [PVD]) in lenalidomide (LEN)-refractory and proteasome inhibitor (PI)-exposed myeloma. J Clin Oncol. 2014;32:Abstract 8589.

13. Wang M, Martin T, Bensinger W, et al. Phase 2 dose-expansion study (PX-171-006) of carfilzomib, lenalidomide, and low-dose dexamethasone in relapsed or progressive multiple myeloma. Blood. 2013;122:3122–8. doi:10.1182/blood-2013-07-511170.

14. Shah JJ, Stadtmauer EA, Abonour R, et al. Carfilzomib, pomalidomide, and dexamethasone for relapsed or refractory myeloma. Blood. 2015;126:2284–90. doi:10.1182/blood-2015-05-643320.

15. Chanan-Khan AA, Kaufman JL, Mehta J, et al. Activity and safety of bortezomib in multiple myeloma patients with advanced renal failure: a multicenter retrospective study. Blood. 2007;109:2604–6. doi:10.1182/blood-2006-09-046409.

16. Tosi P, Zamagni E, Cellini C, et al. Thalidomide alone or in combination with dexamethasone in patients with advanced, relapsed or refractory multiple myeloma and renal failure. Eur J Haematol. 2004;73:98–103. doi:10.1111/j.1600-0609.2004.00272.x.

17. Eriksson T, Höglund P, Turesson I, et al. Pharmacokinetics of thalidomide in patients with impaired renal function and while on and off dialysis. J Pharm Pharmacol. 2003;55:1701–6. doi:10.1211/0022357022241.

18. Rossi AC, Aneja E, Boyer A, et al. Effect of renal and hepatic function on pomalidomide dose in patients with relapsed/refractory multiple myeloma. Blood. 2014;124:4754.

19. Kintzel PE, Dorr RT. Anticancer drug renal toxicity and elimination: dosing guidelines for altered renal function. Cancer Treat Rev. 1995;21:33–64.

20. Bladé J, Sonneveld P, San Miguel JF, et al. Pegylated liposomal doxorubicin plus bortezomib in relapsed or refractory multiple myeloma: efficacy and safety in patients with renal function impairment. Clin Lymphoma Myeloma. 2008;8:352–5. doi:10.3816/CLM.2008.n.051.

21. Owen JS, Melhem M, Passarell JA, et al. Bendamustine pharmacokinetic profile and exposure-response relationships in patients with indolent non-Hodgkin's lymphoma. Cancer Chemother Pharmacol. 2010;66:1039–49. doi:10.1007/s00280-010-1254-8.

22. Sharma S, Witteveen PO, Lolkema MP, et al. A phase I, open-label, multicenter study to evaluate the pharmacokinetics and safety of oral panobinostat in patients with advanced solid tumors and varying degrees of renal function. Cancer Chemother Pharmacol. 2015;75:87–95. doi:10.1007/s00280-014-2612-8.

23. Niesvizky R, Naib T, Christos PJ, et al. Lenalidomide-induced myelosuppression is associated with renal dysfunction: adverse events evaluation of treatment-naïve patients undergoing front-line lenalidomide and dexamethasone therapy. Br J Haematol. 2007;138:640–3. doi:10.1111/j.1365-2141.2007.06698.x.

24. Palumbo A, Bringhen S, Ludwig H, et al. Personalized therapy in multiple myeloma according to patient age and vulnerability: a report of the European Myeloma Network (EMN). Blood. 2011;118:4519–29. doi:10.1182/blood-2011-06-358812.

25. Petrucci MT, Giraldo P, Corradini P, et al. A prospective, international phase 2 study of bortezomib retreatment in patients with relapsed multiple myeloma. Br J Haematol. 2013;160:649–59. doi:10.1111/bjh.12198.

26. Knopf KB, Duh MS, Lafeuille M-H, et al. Meta-analysis of the efficacy and safety of bortezomib re-treatment in patients with multiple myeloma. Clin Lymphoma Myeloma Leuk. 2014;14:380–8. doi:10.1016/j.clml.2014.03.005.

27. Avet-Loiseau H, Attal M, Moreau P, et al. Genetic abnormalities and survival in multiple myeloma: the experience of the Intergroupe Francophone du Myélome. Blood. 2007;109:3489–95. doi:10.1182/blood-2006-08-040410.

28. Avet-Loiseau H, Leleu X, Roussel M, et al. Bortezomib plus dexamethasone induction improves outcome of patients with t(4;14) myeloma but not outcome of patients with del(17p). J Clin Oncol. 2010;28:4630–4. doi:10.1200/JCO.2010.28.3945.

29. Jakubowiak AJ, Siegel DS, Martin T, et al. Treatment outcomes in patients with relapsed and refractory multiple myeloma and high-risk cytogenetics receiving single-agent carfilzomib in the PX-171-003-A1 study. Leukemia. 2013;27:2351–6. doi:10.1038/leu.2013.152.

30. Leleu X, Karlin L, Macro M, et al. Pomalidomide plus low-dose dexamethasone in multiple myeloma with deletion 17p and/or translocation (4;14): IFM 2010-02 trial results. Blood. 2015;125:1411–7. doi:10.1182/blood-2014-11-612069.

31. Moreau P, Masszi T, Grzasko N, et al. Ixazomib, an Investigational Oral Proteasome Inhibitor (PI), in Combination with Lenalidomide and Dexamethasone (IRd), Significantly Extends Progression-Free Survival (PFS) for Patients (Pts) with Relapsed and/or Refractory Multiple Myeloma (RRMM): the phase 3 tourmaline-MM1 study (NCT01564537). Blood. 2015;126:727.

32. Chari A. Novel targets in multiple myeloma. Am J Hematol/Oncol. 2015;11:11–6.

33. Sharman JP, Chmielecki J, Morosini D, et al. Vemurafenib response in 2 patients with post-transplant refractory BRAF V600E-mutated multiple myeloma. Clin Lymphoma Myeloma Leuk. 2014;14:e161–3. doi:10.1016/j.clml.2014.06.004.

34. Chang-Yew Leow C, Gerondakis S, Spencer A. MEK inhibitors as a chemotherapeutic intervention in multiple myeloma. Blood Cancer J. 2013;3:e105. doi:10.1038/bcj.2013.1.

35. Heuck C, Johann D, Walker BA, et al. Characterization of the mutational landscape of multiple myeloma using comprehensive genomic profiling. Blood. 2014;124:3418.

36. Stewart AK, Rajkumar SV, Dimopoulos MA, et al. Carfilzomib, lenalidomide, and dexamethasone for relapsed multiple myeloma. N Engl J Med. 2015;372:142–52. doi:10.1056/NEJMoa1411321.

37. Dimopoulos MA, Moreau P, Palumbo A, et al. Carfilzomib and dexamethasone (Kd) vs bortezomib and dexamethasone (Vd) in patients (pts) with relapsed multiple myeloma (RMM): results from the phase III study ENDEAVOR. J Clin Oncol. 2015;33:Abstract 8509.

38. Papadopoulos KP, Siegel DS, Vesole DH, et al. Phase I study of 30-minute infusion of carfilzomib as single agent or in combination with low-dose dexamethasone in patients with relapsed and/or refractory multiple myeloma. J Clin Oncol. 2015;33:732–9. doi:10.1200/JCO.2013.52.3522.

39. Chari A, Cho HJ, Parekh S, et al. Recapturing disease response: a phase II study of high dose carfilzomib in patients with relapsed or refractory multiple myeloma who have progressed on standard dose carfilzomib. Blood. 2015;126:3051.

40. Kumar SK, Bensinger WI, Zimmerman TM, et al. Phase 1 study of weekly dosing with the investigational oral proteasome inhibitor ixazomib in relapsed/refractory multiple myeloma. Blood. 2014;124:1047–55. doi:10.1182/blood-2014-01-548941.

41. Richardson PG, Baz R, Wang M, et al. Phase 1 study of twice-weekly ixazomib, an oral proteasome inhibitor, in relapsed/refractory multiple myeloma patients. Blood. 2014;124:1038–46. doi:10.1182/blood-2014-01-548826.

42. Voorhees PM, Mulkey F, Hassoun H, et al. Alliance A061202. A phase I/II study of pomalidomide, dexamethasone and ixazomib versus pomalidomide and dexamethasone for patients with multiple myeloma refractory to lenalidomide and proteasome inhibitor based therapy: phase I results. Blood. 2015;126:375.

43. Reu FJ, Valent J, Malek E, et al. A phase I study of ixazomib in combination with panobinostat and dexamethasone in patients with relapsed or refractory multiple myeloma. Blood. 2015;126:4221.

44. San-Miguel JF, Hungria VTM, Yoon S-S, et al. Panobinostat plus bortezomib and dexamethasone versus placebo plus bortezomib and dexamethasone in patients with relapsed or relapsed and refractory multiple myeloma: a multicentre, randomised, double-blind phase 3 trial. Lancet Oncol. 2014;15:1195–206. doi:10.1016/S1470-2045(14)70440-1.

45. Richardson PG, Schlossman RL, Alsina M, et al. PANORAMA 2: panobinostat in combination with bortezomib and dexamethasone in patients with relapsed and bortezomib-refractory myeloma. Blood. 2013;122:2331–7. doi:10.1182/blood-2013-01-481325.

46. Chari A, Cho HJ, Leng S, et al. A phase II study of panobinostat with lenalidomide and weekly dexamethasone in myeloma. Blood. 2015;126:4226.

47. Kaufman JL, Zimmerman T, Rosenbaum CA, et al. Phase I study of the combination of carfilzomib and panobinostat for patients with relapsed and refractory myeloma: a Multiple Myeloma Research Consortium (MMRC) Clinical trial. Blood. 2014;124:32.

48. Larocca A, Montefusco V, Bringhen S, et al. Pomalidomide, cyclophosphamide, and prednisone for relapsed/refractory multiple myeloma: a multicenter phase 1/2 open-label study. Blood. 2013;122:2799–806. doi:10.1182/blood-2013-03-488676.

49. Rossi A, Mark TM, Rodriguez M, et al. Clarithromycin, pomalidomide, and dexamethasone (ClaPD) in relapsed or refractory multiple myeloma. J Clin Oncol. 2012;30:Abstract 8036.

50. Gonsalves WI, Gertz MA, Lacy MQ, et al. Second auto-SCT for treatment of relapsed multiple myeloma. Bone Marrow Transplant. 2013;48:568–73. doi:10.1038/bmt.2012.183.

51. Kortuem KM, Zidich K, Schuster SR, et al. Activity of 129 single-agent drugs in 228 phase I and II clinical trials in multiple myeloma. Clin Lymphoma Myeloma Leuk. 2014;14:284–290. e5. doi:10.1016/j.clml.2013.12.015.

52. Potts BC, Albitar MX, Anderson KC, et al. Marizomib, a proteasome inhibitor for all seasons: preclinical profile and a framework for clinical trials. Curr Cancer Drug Targets. 2011;11:254–84.

53. Richardson PG, Spencer A, Cannell P, et al. Phase 1 clinical evaluation of twice-weekly Marizomib (NPI-0052), a novel proteasome inhibitor, in patients with relapsed/refractory multiple myeloma (MM). Blood. 2011;118:302.

54. Spencer A, Laubach JP, Zonder JA, et al. Phase 1, multicenter, open-label, combination study (NPI-0052-107; NCT02103335) of Pomalidomide (POM), Marizomib (MRZ, NPI-0052), and low-dose dexamethasone (LD-DEX) in patients with relapsed and refractory multiple myeloma. Blood. 2015;126:4220.

55. Jones SS. ACY-1215, a first-in-class selective inhibitor of HDAC6, demonstrates significant synergy with immunomodulatory drugs (IMiDs) in preclinical models of multiple myeloma (MM). Blood. 2013;122:1952.

56. Raje NS, Bensinger W, Cole CE, et al. Ricolinostat (ACY-1215), the first selective HDAC6 inhibitor, combines safely with pomalidomide and dexamethasone and shows promising early results in relapsed-and-refractory myeloma (ACE-MM-102 study). Blood. 2015;126:4228.

57. Vogl DT, Raje NS, Jagannath S, et al. Ricolinostat (ACY-1215), the first selective HDAC6 inhibitor, in combination with bortezomib and dexamethasone in patients with relapsed or relapsed-and-refractory multiple myeloma: phase 1b results (ACY-100 study). Blood. 2015;126:1827.

58. Ocio EM, Richardson PG, Rajkumar SV, et al. New drugs and novel mechanisms of action in multiple myeloma in 2013: a report from the International Myeloma Working Group (IMWG). Leukemia. 2014;28:525–42. doi:10.1038/leu.2013.350.

59. Shah JJ, Zonder J, Cohen A, et al. ARRY-520 shows durable responses in patients with relapsed/refractory multiple myeloma in a phase 1 dose-escalation study. Blood. 2011;118:1860.
60. Lonial S, Shah JJ, Zonder J, et al. Prolonged survival and improved response rates with ARRY-520 in relapsed/refractory multiple myeloma (RRMM) patients with low α-1 acid glycoprotein (AAG) levels: results from a phase 2 study. Blood. 2013;122:285.
61. Chari A, Htut M, Zonder J, et al. A phase 1 study of ARRY-520 with bortezomib (BTZ) and dexamethasone (dex) in relapsed or refractory multiple myeloma (RRMM). Blood. 2013;122:1938.
62. Zonder JA, Usmani S, Scott EC, et al. Phase 2 study of carfilzomib (CFZ) with or without filanesib (FIL) in patients with advanced multiple myeloma (MM). Blood. 2015;126:728.
63. Tai Y-T, Landesman Y, Acharya C, et al. CRM1 inhibition induces tumor cell cytotoxicity and impairs osteoclastogenesis in multiple myeloma: molecular mechanisms and therapeutic implications. Leukemia. 2014;28:155–65. doi:10.1038/leu.2013.115.
64. Chen C, Garzon R, Gutierrez M, et al. Safety, efficacy, and determination of the recommended phase 2 dose for the oral selective inhibitor of nuclear export (SINE) selinexor (KPT-330). Blood. 2015;126:258.
65. Chen CI, Gutierrez M, Siegel DS, et al. Selinexor demonstrates marked synergy with dexamethasone (Sel-Dex) in preclinical models and in patients with heavily pretreated refractory multiple myeloma (MM). Blood. 2014;124:4773.
66. Jakubowiak A, Jasielec J, Rosenbaum CA, et al. Phase 1 MMRC trial of selinexor, carfilzomib (CFZ), and dexamethasone (DEX) in relapsed and relapsed/refractory multiple myeloma (RRMM). Blood. 2015;126:4223.
67. Vij R, Huff CA, Bensinger WI, et al. Ibrutinib, single agent or in combination with dexamethasone, in patients with relapsed or relapsed/refractory multiple myeloma (MM): preliminary phase 2 results. Blood. 2014;124:31.
68. Chari A, Chhabra S, Usmani S, et al. Combination treatment of the bruton's tyrosine kinase inhibitor ibrutinib and carfilzomib in patients with relapsed or relapsed and refractory multiple myeloma: initial results from a multicenter phase 1/2b study. Blood. 2015;126:377.
69. Kumar SK, LaPlant B, Chng WJ, et al. Dinaciclib, a novel CDK inhibitor, demonstrates encouraging single-agent activity in patients with relapsed multiple myeloma. Blood. 2015;125:443–8. doi:10.1182/blood-2014-05-573741.
70. Spencer A, Yoon S-S, Harrison SJ, et al. The novel AKT inhibitor afuresertib shows favorable safety, pharmacokinetics, and clinical activity in multiple myeloma. Blood. 2014;124:2190–5. doi:10.1182/blood-2014-03-559963.
71. Voorhees P, Spencer A, Sutherland HJ, et al. Novel akt inhibitor afuresertib in combination with bortezomib and dexamethasone demonstrates favorable safety profile and significant clinical activity in patients with relapsed/refractory multiple myeloma. Blood. 2013;122:283.
72. Raab MS, Ocio EM, Thomas SK, et al. Phase 1 study update of the novel pan-Pim kinase inhibitor LGH447 in patients with relapsed/refractory multiple myeloma. Blood. 2014;124:301.
73. Lokhorst HM, Plesner T, Gimsing P, et al. Phase I/II dose-escalation study of daratumumab in patients with relapsed or refractory multiple myeloma. J Clin Oncol. 2013;31:Abstract 8512.
74. Lonial S, Weiss BM, Usmani SZ, et al. Phase II study of daratumumab (DARA) monotherapy in patients with ≥ 3 lines of prior therapy or double refractory multiple myeloma (MM): 54767414MMY2002 (Sirius). J Clin Oncol. 2015;33:Abstract LBA8512.
75. Chari A, Satta T, Tayal A, et al. Outcomes and management of red blood cell transfusions in multiple myeloma patients treated with daratumumab. Blood. 2015;126:3571.
76. Plesner T, Arkenau H-T, Gimsing P, et al. Daratumumab in combination with lenalidomide and dexamethasone in patients with relapsed or relapsed and refractory multiple myeloma: updated results of a phase 1/2 study (GEN503). Blood. 2015;126:507.
77. Chari A, Lonial S, Suvannasankha A, et al. Open-label, multicenter, phase 1b study of daratumumab in combination with pomalidomide and dexamethasone in patients with at least 2 lines of prior therapy and relapsed or relapsed and refractory multiple myeloma. Blood. 2015;126:508.
78. Lonial S, Dimopoulos M, Palumbo A, et al. Elotuzumab therapy for relapsed or refractory multiple myeloma. N Engl J Med. 2015;373:621–31. doi:10.1056/NEJMoa1505654.

79. Palumbo A, Offidani M, Pégourie B, et al. Elotuzumab plus bortezomib and dexamethasone versus bortezomib and dexamethasone in patients with relapsed/refractory multiple myeloma: 2-year follow-up. Blood. 2015;126:510.
80. Martin T, Richter J, Vij R, et al. A dose finding phase II trial of isatuximab (SAR650984, anti-CD38 mAb) as a single agent in relapsed/refractory multiple myeloma. Blood. 2015;126:509.
81. Kelly KR, Chanan-Khan A, Heffner LT, et al. Indatuximab ravtansine (BT062) in combination with lenalidomide and low-dose dexamethasone in patients with relapsed and/or refractory multiple myeloma: clinical activity in patients already exposed to lenalidomide and bortezomib. Blood. 2014;124:4736.
82. Rosenblatt J, Vasir B, Uhl L, et al. Vaccination with dendritic cell/tumor fusion cells results in cellular and humoral antitumor immune responses in patients with multiple myeloma. Blood. 2011;117:393–402. doi:10.1182/blood-2010-04-277137.
83. Rosenblatt J, Avivi I, Vasir B, et al. Vaccination with dendritic cell/tumor fusions following autologous stem cell transplant induces immunologic and clinical responses in multiple myeloma patients. Clin Cancer Res. 2013;19:3640–8. doi:10.1158/1078-0432.CCR-13-0282.
84. Luptakova K, Rosenblatt J, Glotzbecker B, et al. Lenalidomide enhances anti-myeloma cellular immunity. Cancer Immunol Immunother. 2013;62:39–49. doi:10.1007/s00262-012-1308-3.
85. Bensinger WI, Buckner CD, Anasetti C, et al. Allogeneic marrow transplantation for multiple myeloma: an analysis of risk factors on outcome. Blood. 1996;88:2787–93.
86. Smith E, Devlin SM, Kosuri S, et al. CD34-selected allogeneic hematopoietic stem cell transplantation for patients with relapsed, high-risk multiple myeloma, Biol Blood Marrow Transplant. 2015. doi:10.1016/j.bbmt.2015.08.025.
87. Brahmer JR, Tykodi SS, Chow LQM, et al. Safety and activity of anti-PD-L1 antibody in patients with advanced cancer. N Engl J Med. 2012;366:2455–65. doi:10.1056/NEJMoa1200694.
88. Topalian SL, Hodi FS, Brahmer JR, et al. Safety, activity, and immune correlates of anti-PD-1 antibody in cancer. N Engl J Med. 2012;366:2443–54. doi:10.1056/NEJMoa1200690.
89. San Miguel J, Mateos M-V, Shah JJ, et al. Pembrolizumab in combination with lenalidomide and low-dose dexamethasone for relapsed/refractory multiple myeloma (RRMM): keynote-023. Blood. 2015;126:505.
90. Badros AZ, Kocoglu MH, Ma N, et al. A phase II study of anti PD-1 antibody pembrolizumab, pomalidomide and dexamethasone in patients with relapsed/refractory multiple myeloma (RRMM). Blood. 2015;126:506.
91. Garfall AL, Maus MV, Hwang W-T, et al. Chimeric antigen receptor T cells against CD19 for multiple myeloma. N Engl J Med. 2015;373:1040–7. doi:10.1056/NEJMoa1504542.
92. Ali SA, Shi V, Wang M, et al. Remissions of multiple myeloma during a first-in-humans clinical trial of T cells expressing an anti-B-cell maturation antigen chimeric antigen receptor. Blood. 2015;126:LBA–1–LBA–1.
93. Krishnan A, Pasquini MC, Logan B, et al. Autologous haemopoietic stem-cell transplantation followed by allogeneic or autologous haemopoietic stem-cell transplantation in patients with multiple myeloma (BMT CTN 0102): a phase 3 biological assignment trial. Lancet Oncol. 2011;12:1195–203. doi:10.1016/S1470-2045(11)70243-1.

Plasma Cell Leukemia

7

Nisha S. Joseph, Amarendra K. Neppalli, and Ajay K. Nooka

7.1 Introduction

Plasma cell leukemia is a rare and an aggressive variant of multiple myeloma that is characterized by the presence of circulating plasma cells in peripheral blood. By the International Myeloma Working Group (IMWG) consensus statement on the diagnostic criteria, existence of $\geq 20\%$ and/or an absolute number of $\geq 2 \times 10^9$/L circulating plasma cells are required to confirm the diagnosis of PCL [1]. Nevertheless, the presence of circulating plasma cells on conventional morphology by itself confers a poorer risk with survival outcomes akin to patients with PCL [2]. This more likely represents the extramedullary presentation of myeloma, suggesting that these resistant plasma cells are capable of survival independent of the bone marrow microenvironment and clinically present as an aggressive plasma cell neoplasm unresponsive to most conventional therapies. For the same reason, certain groups have proposed to lower the threshold of the circulating plasma cells to fit the criteria of diagnosis of PCL and suggested the presence of circulating plasma cells be treated as high-risk myeloma.

N.S. Joseph • A.K. Nooka (✉)
Department of Hematology and Oncology, Winship Cancer Institute, Emory University, Atlanta, GA 30345, USA
e-mail: anooka@emory.edu

A.K. Neppalli
Department of Medicine, Medical University of South Carolina, Charleston, SC 29425, USA

© Springer International Publishing AG 2018
S.Z. Usmani, A.K. Nooka (eds.), *Personalized Therapy for Multiple Myeloma*,
https://doi.org/10.1007/978-3-319-61872-2_7

7.2 Prognosis

With the existing definition, PCL represents approximately 2–4% of all MM diagnoses and exists in two forms: primary PCL (pPCL, 60–70% of cases) which presents de novo and secondary PCL (sPCL, 30–40% of cases) which represents leukemic transformation in patients with a previously diagnosed plasma cell dyscrasia and evolves as a terminal event. If the circulating plasma cells in the diagnostic criteria are lowered to 2%, the incidence could account for as high as 14% [2]. The disease traditionally portends a poor outcome, and the median survival for pPCL is less than 1 year with conventional treatment and for sPCL less than 3 months. A population-based analysis using the surveillance, epidemiology, and end results (SEER) registry demonstrated the modest improvement in survival for pPCL based on periods of diagnosis. Survival from the time period 2006–2009 vs. 2001–2005 vs. 1996–2000 vs. 1973–1995 was 12 vs. 4 vs. 6 vs. 5 months, respectively ($P = 0.001$), suggesting that use of better non-chemotherapeutic strategies could result in improved outcomes for pPCL [3].

7.3 Clinical Presentation

In general, both pPCL and sPCL exhibit more aggressive clinical presentations than myeloma, including a higher tumor burden. Usually seen among younger patients, pPCL exhibits remarkable heterogeneity and high mutational burden. Though both phenotypes have overlapping genetic abnormalities, these are not identical. The prevalence of high-risk chromosomal abnormalities, such as del(17p), del(1p21), and *MYC* translocations or amplifications, is markedly higher compared with newly diagnosed myeloma [4, 5]. Activating *K-RAS* and *N-RAS* mutations are frequently observed in pPCL [6]. The incidence of hyperdiploidy is very uncommon in pPCL [4], while sPCL patients like myeloma patients may present with hyperdiploidy. In pPCL the IgH translocations are exclusively targeted at 11q13 (*CCND1*)—a nonhyperdiploid t(11;14) (q13;q32) [4]—while in sPCL, the IgH translocations can present as t(11;14), t(4;14), or t (14;16) similar to the spectrum of translocations observed in myeloma [5]. Clinically, high symptom burden (anemia, renal dysfunction, hypercalcemia) leading to disease-related morbidity is more common among pPCL patients. Interestingly, the presence of lytic bone lesions is lower in pPCL patients than that observed in myeloma. In contrast, the higher prevalence of advanced bone disease in sPCL probably represents the terminal stage of preceding myeloma, where advanced bone disease is more common [5]. pPCL patients may exhibit a higher prevalence of extramedullary involvement of the liver, spleen, lymph nodes, pleural effusions, neurological deficits due to central nervous system involvement, and palpable extramedullary soft-tissue plasmacytomas. Laboratory studies demonstrate elevated LDH and β2-microglobulin indicative of higher tumor burden and high proliferation index.

7.4   Diagnostic Evaluation for PCL

As is necessary for myeloma, a thorough medical history and physical examination to evaluate for extramedullary involvement are of utmost importance for timely diagnosis. A complete blood count with manual differential, with specific examination of the peripheral blood smear for plasma cells, is needed. A comprehensive metabolic panel (BUN, creatinine, calcium), liver function panel (albumin, total protein, transaminases, bilirubin), and tumor lysis parameters (LDH, uric acid, calcium, phosphate, potassium) are needed. Other myeloma initial staging studies such as β2-microglobulin and albumin (for ISS staging), serum protein electrophoresis, immunofixation, serum-free light chain analysis, immunophenotyping, 24-h urine collection for total protein estimation, electrophoresis, and immunofixation are required. Bone marrow aspirate and biopsy and cytogenetic analysis by FISH focused on del(17p13), del(13q), del(1p21), amp l(1q21), t(11;14), t(4;14), and t(14;16) are strongly recommended. Skeletal survey is routinely indicated.

Additional investigations may be useful where there is clinical suspicion for other organ involvements. Constant evaluation for CNS symptoms is mandatory. A low threshold should be adopted for obtaining a lumbar puncture if there is suspicion for leptomeningeal involvement. Utilizing the more sensitive imaging techniques such as MRI for evaluation of cord compression and using 18F-FDG-PET/CT for evaluation of extramedullary involvement are clinically indicated. HLA typing for younger patients should be done as a part of initial workup, in case an allogeneic stem cell transplant (SCT) is considered in the future.

7.5   Therapeutic Options for PCL

Given the rarity of its presentation, there are no standard therapeutic strategies that have been proven to be superior over the other treatments. However, in the recent era of availability of novel agents, the increasing utilization of SCT small series with few patients has demonstrated the benefits of combining these strategies in attaining somewhat better outcomes.

To date, there have been only two prospective clinical trials published for the initial treatment of pPCL. The first trial evaluated a combination of lenalidomide and low-dose dexamethasone (Rd) as initial therapy among pPCL patients. Per protocol, responders after four cycles will move forward with SCT, and responding transplant-ineligible patients continue four more cycles followed by maintenance cycles of dose-reduced lenalidomide until relapse. With an overall response rate (ORR) of 73.9% (39% ≥ VGPR), at a median follow-up of 34 months, median progression-free survival (PFS) was 14 months, and median overall survival (OS) was 28 months [7]. PFS was 21 months vs. 10 months for SCT eligible vs. non-eligible patients, and OS also benefitted the SCT eligible patients as well. The second prospective trial evaluated bortezomib, doxorubicin, cyclophosphamide, and dexamethasone induction followed by SCT for pPCL [8]. The ORR was 69% (36% ≥ VGPR); 25 patients underwent SCT, and 1 patient received a syngeneic transplant. At 3 months' post-SCT, 16 patients underwent tandem SCT with reduced intensity conditioning (RIC) allogeneic SCT (RIC-allo-SCT). At a median follow-up of 28.7 months, the median PFS was 15.1 months, and the median OS was 36.3 months. Though a case was made for RIC-allo-SCT, these results were almost comparable with the prior trial using Rd followed by SCT albeit less toxicity. While the median OS is 36.3 months for patients who effectively underwent first transplant ($n = 26$), the median OS was 10.5 months in patients with primary refractory disease. This uniform theme in both trials with high early progression rates among close to 25% of patients suggests that an effective up-front regimen using CD38 monoclonal antibody combinations could potentially counter the biologically aggressive disease process.

Several other retrospective analyses both using registry data and using data from single-institution analyses suggested that combining novel agents, predominantly bortezomib-based regimens, and transplant led to improved outcomes (Table 7.1) The EBMT group reported a median PFS and OS significantly shorter in pPCL relative to myeloma patients (PFS, 14.3 months vs. 27.4 months; OS, 25.7 months vs. 62.3 months, respectively; both $p = 0.000$), despite complete response (CR) rates before and after SCT which were higher in the pPCL group. These results could be due to the higher transplant-related mortality (TRM) and short duration of the posttransplant response in pPCL group [9]. In contrast, in a retrospective analysis performed by the CIBMTR, the authors did not find inferior post-SCT survival in pPCL compared with myeloma. A PFS and OS at 3 years in the pPCL group of 34% and 64%, respectively, were reported. The authors also described a trend toward an OS benefit for the tandem SCT instead of a single transplant [10]. Considering the differing years of SCT and the lack of information regarding the induction regimen in the EBMT analysis and the lack of information on the use of maintenance therapy in the CIBMTR study, definitive conclusions cannot be drawn. However, both analyses suggested that the poor clinical outcomes of PCL seemed to be ameliorated by utilizing the SCT approach. These results align with the data form other series reporting a median OS of 34 months among pPCL patients that received SCT compared to OS of 11 months among patients treated with chemotherapy alone [5].

Bortezomib has recently been demonstrated to have clinical activity in both pPCL and sPCL, either in combination or sequentially after other chemotherapies. In a large retrospective analysis from the Italian GIMEMA MM Working Party, 29 patients with pPCL received different chemotherapy combinations containing bortezomib as frontline therapy and reported promising results in terms of ORR (79%), PFS, and OS (2-year PFS and OS, 40% and 55%, respectively). The best outcomes, however, were observed in patients who received SCT as consolidation after induction, whereas other patients had a shorter period of remission [11]. The same group showed, in a retrospective analysis including patients with pPCL and sPCL treated with bortezomib alone or in association with other drugs, a median PFS and OS of

Table 7.1 Clinical outcomes of plasma cell leukemia from selected studies

Study	Phase	pPCL	sPCL	Characteristics	Median age (year)	PFS	OS (m)	Comments
Musto [7]	Prospective trial	23		Rd	60	14 m	28 m	Median f/u 34 m; ORR, 73.9%; ≥ VGPR, 39%; OS favored SCT eligible patients
Royer [8]	Prospective trial	40		VCDD	57	15.1 m	36.3 m	Median f/u 28.7 m; ORR, 69%; ≥ VGPR, 59%; SCT 26 pts. (65%)
Drake [9]	Retrospective registry	272			55	14.3 m	25.7 m	OS for pts. with pPCL in < CR, 21 m; ≥CR, 30 m
Mahindra [10]	Retrospective registry	147		97 (auto) 50 (allo)	56 (auto) 48 (allo)	34% (3-year PFS) 20% (3-year PFS)	64% (3-year OS) 39% (3-year OS)	Median f/u, 38 m; 3-year PFS, 36% (single), 37% (tandem); 3-year OS, 56% (single), 84% (tandem)
Avet-Loiseau [15]	Retrospective working group	70		46 pts. (<65) Del (17) p, 20%	60		16 m	Median OS, 31 m for younger pts. treated intensively; no benefit for novel agents (BTZ)
D'Arena [11]	Retrospective working group	29		BTZ regimens	62	40% (2-year PFS)	55% (2-year OS)	Median f/u, 24 m; CR 28%
Katodritou [17]	Retrospective working group	25	17	BTZ regimens	66 (pPCL) 64 (sPCL)	13 m (pPCL)	16 m (pPCL) 2 m (sPCL)	Median f/u 51 m; OS with BTZ pPCL vs. sPCL, 18 m vs. 7 m

(continued)

Table 7.1 (continued)

Study	Phase	pPCL	sPCL	Characteristics	Median age (year)	PFS	OS (m)	Comments
Iriuchishima [20]	Retrospective working group	38		Novel regimens, 61%		2.85 years		OS favored pts. receiving maintenance therapy
Pagano [21]	Retrospective multi-institution	73		SCT, 23 (31%)			12.6 m	OS, SCT vs. non-SCT, 38 m vs. 9.1 m; BTZ/thal use HR 0.47
Lebovic [13]	Retrospective single institution	13	12	19 (auto) 6 (allo)			23.6 m	OS with BTZ vs. no BTZ, 28.4 m vs. 4 m
Usmani [14]	Retrospective single institution	27		TT1, TT2, TT3 protocols		10 m	20 m	CR duration 16 m, improved with BTZ/thal; pPCL were overrepresented in the MF and CD1 molecular subgroups
Tiedemann [5]	Retrospective single institution	41	39	pPCL (21 pts., chemo combos, 20 MP)	54.5 (pPCL) 65.7 (sPCL)		11.2 m (pPCL) 1.3 m (sPCL)	OS for MP vs. chemo combos (VAD, VBMCP), 4.1 m vs. 15.4 m; OS favored SCT patients
Nooka [16]	Retrospective single institution	22	6	95% SCT (pPCL)		66% (3-year PFS) (pPCL) 3 m (sPCL)	73% (4-year OS) (pPCL) 3 m (sPCL)	PFS RVD maintenance vs. no, 38 m vs. 15 m; 3-year OS: RVD maintenance vs. no, 100% vs. 67%
Musto [12]	Retrospective single institution	8	4	BTZ regimens	61.2	8 m	12 m	

M months; *OS* overall survival; *pPCL* primary plasma cell leukemia; *sPCL* secondary plasma cell leukemia; *PFS* progression-free survival; *OS* overall survival; *auto* autotransplant; *allo* allotransplant; *BTZ* bortezomib; *Rd* lenalidomide and low-dose dexamethasone; *VCDD* bortezomib, doxorubicin, cyclophosphamide, and dexamethasone; *MP* melphalan and prednisone; *RVD* lenalidomide, bortezomib, and dexamethasone; *HR* hazard ratio

8 and 12 months, respectively. The median PFS and OS for pPCL were not reached after 21 months of follow-up [12]. The efficacy of the proteasome inhibitors has also been confirmed in other analyses. Patients that received bortezomib had superior outcomes compared to the bortezomib-naïve patients (OS, 28.4 months vs. 4 months; $p = 0.001$) [13]. In contrast, Usmani et al. reported their experience on pPCL in a large series of 1474 patients with myeloma enrolled in total therapy protocols or in a TT3-like approach. The presence of pPCL was associated with a significantly shorter PFS and OS (10 months and 20 months, respectively); no difference in outcome was seen with the addition of bortezomib in PCL patients, and the CR rates in the two groups were the same [14]. In the same vein, the IFM group didn't observe survival differences between patients treated with bortezomib and those treated with old drugs [15].

In this context, our institutional data of 28 patients sheds light on the benefits of an optimal induction regimen and the benefits of an intense maintenance approach. Majority received a bortezomib-based induction regimen followed by immediate SCT and lenalidomide, bortezomib, and dexamethasone (RVD) maintenance. The PFS rate was 66% at 3 years, and OS rate was 73% at 4 years [16]. Median PFS for patients receiving maintenance with RVD vs. no RVD maintenance was 38 vs. 15 months ($p = 0.004$). Three-year OS for patients on RVD maintenance vs. no maintenance was 100% vs. 67%; $p = 0.018$. Achieving ≥VGPR vs. <VGPR post-SCT (PFS, 38 vs. 14 months, $p = 0.002$, and OS, 49 vs. 26 months, $p = 0.037$) strongly predicted outcomes.

Very few studies have evaluated the exclusive outcomes of sPCL. The median PFS and OS in this subgroup of patients are less than 3 months [5, 16, 17]. Newer treatment options incorporating the monoclonal antibody combinations and other immune approaches are much needed in treating these patients.

Despite the use of SCT and the introduction of new drugs, PCL remains a highly resistant disease characterized by rapid progressions and shorter durations of remission. Especially in this group of patients, the improvement in outcomes is less evident compared to other high-risk myeloma patients. Recognizing the limitations in the lack of huge body of evidence in the PCL patients, from the available literature, SCT can improve the outcomes in pPCL (may not be as effective as in myeloma patients). While no definitive conclusions can be drawn regarding the superiority of one induction regimen over the other, using a triplet regimen such as RVD, similar to the myeloma, would be optimal [18, 19]. Most studies that have demonstrated significant improvement in OS for pPCL patients used maintenance therapy. Based on the available literature, it is very clear that the goal of treating the pPCL patients should be aimed to attain the best depth of response and maintain the response utilizing other modalities of SCT and maintenance approaches. As shown by our group previously, using an effective PI/IMiD induction regimen followed by SCT and consolidation/maintenance with PI/IMiD combinations could be the most optimal strategy to improve depth of response, maintain remission, and prolong survival for this group of patients (Fig. 7.1).

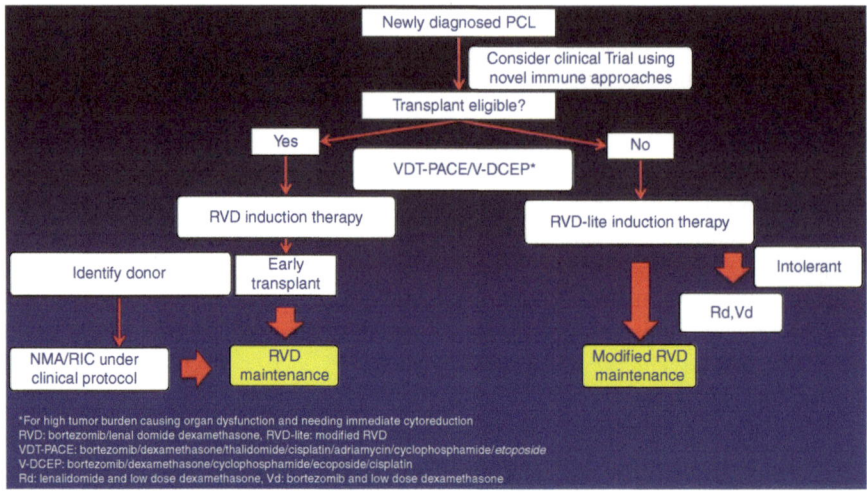

Fig. 7.1 Algorithm for treating plasma cell leukemia

References

1. Fernandez de Larrea C, et al. Plasma cell leukemia: consensus statement on diagnostic requirements, response criteria and treatment recommendations by the International Myeloma Working Group. Leukemia. 2013;27(4):780–91.
2. An G, et al. Multiple myeloma patients with low proportion of circulating plasma cells had similar survival with primary plasma cell leukemia patients. Ann Hematol. 2015;94(2):257–64.
3. Gonsalves WI, et al. Trends in survival of patients with primary plasma cell leukemia: a population-based analysis. Blood. 2014;124(6):907–12.
4. Avet-Loiseau H, et al. Cytogenetic, interphase, and multicolor fluorescence in situ hybridization analyses in primary plasma cell leukemia: a study of 40 patients at diagnosis, on behalf of the Intergroupe Francophone du Myelome and the Groupe Francais de Cytogenetique Hematologique. Blood. 2001;97(3):822–5.
5. Tiedemann RE, et al. Genetic aberrations and survival in plasma cell leukemia. Leukemia. 2008;22(5):1044–52.
6. Bezieau S, et al. High incidence of N and K-Ras activating mutations in multiple myeloma and primary plasma cell leukemia at diagnosis. Hum Mutat. 2001;18(3):212–24.
7. Musto P, et al. Lenalidomide and low-dose dexamethasone for newly diagnosed primary plasma cell leukemia. Leukemia. 2014;28(1):222–5.
8. Royer B, et al. Bortezomib, doxorubicin, cyclophosphamide, dexamethasone induction followed by stem cell transplantation for primary plasma cell leukemia: a prospective phase II study of the Intergroupe Francophone du Myelome. J Clin Oncol. 2016;34(18):2125–32.
9. Drake MB, et al. Primary plasma cell leukemia and autologous stem cell transplantation. Haematologica. 2010;95(5):804–9.
10. Mahindra A, et al. Hematopoietic cell transplantation for primary plasma cell leukemia: results from the Center for International Blood and Marrow Transplant Research. Leukemia. 2012;26(5):1091–7.
11. D'Arena G, et al. Frontline chemotherapy with bortezomib-containing combinations improves response rate and survival in primary plasma cell leukemia: a retrospective study from GIMEMA Multiple Myeloma Working Party. Ann Oncol. 2012;23(6):1499–502.

12. Musto P, et al. Efficacy and safety of bortezomib in patients with plasma cell leukemia. Cancer. 2007;109(11):2285–90.
13. Lebovic D, et al. Clinical outcomes of patients with plasma cell leukemia in the era of novel therapies and hematopoietic stem cell transplantation strategies: a single-institution experience. Clin Lymphoma Myeloma Leuk. 2011;11(6):507–11.
14. Usmani SZ, et al. Primary plasma cell leukemia: clinical and laboratory presentation, gene-expression profiling and clinical outcome with Total Therapy protocols. Leukemia. 2012;26(11):2398–405.
15. Avet-Loiseau H, et al. Cytogenetic and therapeutic characterization of primary plasma cell leukemia: the IFM experience. Leukemia. 2012;26(1):158–9.
16. Nooka AK, et al. Plasma cell leukemia: sustained responses are possible with innovative treatment strategies haematologica 2012. Leukemia. 97(s1):1516.
17. Katodritou E, et al. Treatment with bortezomib-based regimens improves overall response and predicts for survival in patients with primary or secondary plasma cell leukemia: analysis of the Greek myeloma study group. Am J Hematol. 2014;89(2):145–50.
18. Gozzetti A, et al. Efficacy of bortezomib, lenalidomide and dexamethasone (VRD) in secondary plasma cell leukaemia. Br J Haematol. 2012;157(4):497–8.
19. Durie BG, et al. Bortezomib with lenalidomide and dexamethasone versus lenalidomide and dexamethasone alone in patients with newly diagnosed myeloma without intent for immediate autologous stem-cell transplant (SWOG S0777): a randomised, open-label, phase 3 trial. Lancet. 2017;389(10068):519–27.
20. Iriuchishima H, et al. Primary plasma cell leukemia in the era of novel agents: a multicenter study of the japanese society of myeloma. Acta Haematol. 2016;135(2):113–21.
21. Pagano L, et al. Primary plasma cell leukemia: a retrospective multicenter study of 73 patients. Ann Oncol. 2011;22(7):1628–35.

Practical Considerations for Bone Health in Multiple Myeloma

Evangelos Terpos and Nikolaos Kanellias

8.1 Introduction

Multiple myeloma (MM) is a common hematological malignancy characterized by the accumulation of abnormal plasma cells in the bone marrow. Even though survival has been improved after the introduction of novel agents [1, 2], MM remains an incurable plasma-cell malignancy [3, 4]. MM is characterized by osteolytic bone disease due to an elevated function of osteoclasts which is not balanced by a comparable elevation of osteoblast function [5–7]. Osteolytic lesions are detected in 70–80% of patients at diagnosis and increase the risk for skeletal-related events (SREs) (pathologic fractures, spinal cord compression (SCC), requirement for surgery or palliative radiotherapy to bone). SREs have a serious impact on the quality of life (QoL) and survival of MM patients and affect both clinical and economic aspects of their life [8–13]. The novel International Myeloma Working Group (IMWG) criteria for the diagnosis of symptomatic MM have revealed the value of modern imaging for the management of MM patients, as they include (1) the presence at least one lytic lesion detected not only by conventional radiography but also by computed tomography (CT), whole-body low-dose CT (WBLDCT) or positron emission tomography/CT (PET-CT) and (2) the presence of >1 focal bone marrow lesions on magnetic resonance imaging (MRI) studies [14]. Furthermore, novel imaging techniques, such as MRI and PET-CT, provide prognostic information and have been recently proven of value, for the better definition of response to antimyeloma therapy. Bisphosphonates (BPs) are the cornerstone of therapeutic management of myeloma bone disease, offering considerable benefit in preventing or delaying skeletal-related events and relieving pain [15]. This chapter reviews the latest available details of imaging and treatment of myeloma-related bone disease.

E. Terpos (✉) • N. Kanellias
Department of Clinical Therapeutics, National and Kapodistrian University of Athens,
School of Medicine, Athens, Greece
e-mail: eterpos@hotmail.com

© Springer International Publishing AG 2018   131
S.Z. Usmani, A.K. Nooka (eds.), *Personalized Therapy for Multiple Myeloma*,
https://doi.org/10.1007/978-3-319-61872-2_8

8.2   Pathophysiology of Multiple Myeloma Bone Disease

In the adult skeleton, skeletal integrity is coordinated by the synchronized activity of three cell types. Osteoblasts create new bone matrix, osteoclasts are responsible for bone resorption, and osteocytes regulate bone turnover. In MM patients, bone disease is the result of an uncoupling in bone remodeling. It consists of an increase in the osteoclast-mediated bone resorption, which is combined with suppression in the osteoblast, mediated bone mineralization, and defects on osteocyte functions [16]. Until today, several direct and indirect interactions between myeloma cells and cells of the bone marrow microenvironment have been recognized. The fact that osteolytic lesions occur close to MM cells suggests that factors secreted by tumor cells lead to direct stimulation of osteoclast-mediated bone resorption and inhibition of osteoblast-mediated bone formation [6]. In addition to that, the increased bone resorptive progress leads to the release of growth factors that increase the growth of MM cells, leading to a vicious cycle of tumor expansion and bone destruction. Apart from that, interactions via adhesion between MM cells and bone marrow cells result in the production of factors that promote angiogenesis and make the myeloma cells resistant to chemotherapy [17, 18]. The biologic pathway of the receptor activator of nuclear factor-kappa B (RANK), its ligand (RANKL), and osteoprotegerin (OPG) which is the decoy receptor of RANKL is of major importance for the increased osteoclast activity observed in MM. Myeloma cells disrupt the balance between RANKL and OPG by increasing the expression of RANKL and decreasing the expression of OPG. The resulting increase in RANKL favors the formation and activation of osteoclasts, leading to increased bone resorption [19, 20]. More recently, activin A has been implicated in MM bone disease, through stimulating RANK expression and inducing osteoclastogenesis [21, 22]. In addition to their stimulatory effect on osteoclasts, myeloma cells have been shown to suppress bone formation [23]. The Wingless-type (Wnt) signaling pathway is one pathway that has been shown to play a key role in osteoblast differentiation and has been implicated in osteoblast suppression in myeloma. The Wnt signaling inhibitors dickkopf-1 (Dkk-1) and sclerostin are secreted by myeloma cells and have been found to be increased in the serum of myeloma patients, leading to the block of osteoblast differentiation and activity [24–27]. Soluble frizzle-related protein-2 (sFRP-2), another inhibitor of Wnt signaling, has also been implicated in suppression of bone formation in myeloma [28]. Although the circulating levels of the above molecules and mainly of sclerostin have not been found to be elevated in myeloma patients in all published studies, the importance of Wnt inhibition in the biology of myeloma-related bone disease is undoubted.

8.3   Imaging for the Diagnosis of Multiple Myeloma Bone Disease

The imaging techniques used for the diagnosis of multiple myeloma bone disease are:

- Whole-body X-rays (WBXR)
- Whole-body CT (WBCT)

- Magnetic resonance imaging (MRI)
- PET-CT

8.4 Whole-Body X-rays (WBXR)

Conventional radiography has been widely used for the identification of osteolytic lesions both at diagnosis and during the course of the disease. The "skeletal survey" (whole-body X-rays (WBXR)) at diagnosis should include plain radiographs of the whole skeleton (anteroposterior and lateral views of the skull posteroanterior view of the chest; anteroposterior and lateral views of the thoracic lumbar and cervical spine (including an open mouth view), humeri, and femora; and anteroposterior view of the pelvis) [29]. In addition, symptomatic areas should also be specifically visualized. Osteolytic lesions have the typical appearance of "punched-out" lesions with absence of reactive sclerosis and are more common in the vertebrae, ribs, skull, and pelvis [30]. Although the WBXR was the standard of care for many years, it has several limitations: (1) for a lytic lesion to become apparent, >30% loss of trabecular bone must occur; (2) difficulty of assessment of certain areas, such as the pelvis and the spine; (3) limitations in the detection of lytic lesion response to antimyeloma therapy because of delayed evidence of healing; (4) reduced specificity for the differential diagnosis of myeloma-related versus benign fracture (very important, particularly in cases of new vertebral compression fractures in the absence of other criteria of relapse); (5) observer dependency (there is very low reproducibility among centers; higher number of osteolytic lesions detected in academic vs. non-academic centers); and (6) prolonged study length, often not tolerable from patients in severe pain [29, 30]. Thus, the development of novel imaging methods has led to the replacement of WBXR by more advanced techniques, such as the WBLDCT in many European centers or by PET-CT in the USA.

8.5 Whole-Body Low-Dose CT (WBLDCT)

WBLDCT was introduced to allow the detection of osteolytic lesions in the whole skeleton with high accuracy, no need for contrast agents and low radiation dose compared to standard CT (two- to threefold lower radiation dose vs. conventional CT) [31, 32]. In several studies, WBLDCT was found to be superior to WBXR for the detection of osteolytic lesions [31, 33–37]. In one of the largest studies staging myeloma patients, 61% of patients with normal WBXR had more than one osteolytic lesions on WBLDCT [36]. According to the latest criteria for symptomatic myeloma, these patients should receive therapy. In the same study, the total number of lesions detected by WBLDCT was 968 vs. 248 for WBXR ($p < 0.001$). The only limitation of this study was its retrospective origin [36]. In a more recent prospective study, which included 52 myeloma patients at diagnosis, WBLDCT revealed osteolyses in 12 patients (23%) with negative WBXR and proved to be more sensitive than WBXR mainly in the axial skeleton ($p < 0.001$). WBLDCT was superior in the detection of lesions in patients with osteopenia and osteoporosis [37].

In total WBLDCT advantages over WBXR include (1) superior diagnostic sensitivity for depiction of osteolytic lesions, especially in areas where the WBXR detection rate is low, i.e., pelvis and spine; (2) superiority in estimating fracture risk and bone instability; (3) duration of the examination, which is ≤5 min, an important issue for patients in extreme pain; (4) production of higher-quality 3D high-resolution images for planning biopsies and therapeutic interventions; and finally (5) demonstration of unsuspected manifestations of myeloma or other disease, especially in the lungs and kidneys (33% in the study by Wolf et al.; 37, 31–37). Major disadvantages of WBLDCT include increased length of time required for radiologists to report their findings, lack of availability in several centers [14, 31], and lack of specificity for the differential diagnosis between malignant and osteoporotic fractures, despite improvements during the last years [38]. Furthermore, although exposure to radiation is much lower compared to standard CT, it continues to be higher than WBXR: mean dose of WBLDCT is approximately 3.6 and 2.8 mSv for females and males, respectively, versus 1.2 mSv for WBXR [39]. Nevertheless, the higher diagnostic accuracy of the WBLDCT and patient comfort is particularly important for the elderly, and often suffering group renders the dose/quality ratio favorable for WBLDCT. For these reasons, the European Myeloma Network has suggested that WBLDCT should replace conventional radiography as the standard imaging technique for evaluation of bone disease in MM, where available [40].

8.6 Magnetic Resonance Imaging

Techniques. Several MRI techniques have been developed for the assessment of the bone marrow involvement in MM. Conventional MRI protocols include T1-weighted, T2-weighted with fat suppression, short time inversion recovery (STIR), and gadolinium T1-weighted with fat suppression [41]. Myeloma lesions show typically a low signal intensity on T1-weighted images, a high signal intensity on T2-weighted and STIR images, and often enhancement on gadolinium-enhanced images [42, 43].

Limitations of MRI are the prolonged acquisition time, availability issues the high cost, the exclusion of patients with metal devices in their body, the difficulties in cases of claustrophobic patients, and the limited field of view. To override these restrictions, a Whole body MRI (WB-MRI) methodology, which does not usually require contrast infusion, was developed. The time of WB-MRI is approximately 45 min. Although of interest, this newer technique is not yet widely employed.

All above MRI methods use MRI exquisite contrast and spatial resolution for the depiction of the WB anatomy and specific tissue composition in details.

Novel MRI techniques include diffusion-weighted imaging, dynamic contrast-enhanced MRI, and PET-MRI.

A novel and promising MRI sequence is the diffusion-weighted imaging (DWI-MRI) which derives its contrast mainly from differences in the diffusivity of water molecules in the tissue environment. This functional technique demonstrates alterations in intra- and extracellular water content from disruption of the transmembrane water flux that are visible before identified changes on the morphologic routine sequences [44–46]. DWI-MRI uses the calculation of apparent diffusion coefficient (ADC) values to better evaluate myeloma burden and MRI infiltration patterns [47, 48]. DWI can be used to detect regions with bone marrow infiltration for both diagnosis and monitoring treatment response [49], because ADC values are higher in MM patients at diagnosis, compared with patients in remission 20 weeks after initiation of treatment [50]. In MM patients, the ADC was reproducible [51] and correlated with bone marrow cellularity and microvessel density (MVD) [52]. One disadvantage of DWI is that the ADC is not exclusively influenced by diffusion but also by perfusion. However, improved sequences are under development to differentiate both influences [53]. DWI-MRI was found superior to WBXR for the detection of bone involvement in 20 patients with relapsed/refractory MM in all areas of the skeleton except of the skull, where both examinations had equal sensitivity [54]. In another small study with 24 myeloma patients (both treated and untreated), DWI-MRI was found more sensitive than F18-fluorodeoxyglucose (FDG)-PET in the detection of myeloma lesions [55]. In a recent study, 17 patients were evaluated with DWI-MRI and FDG-PET-CT, and the findings were compared with bone marrow biopsy data. In all studied regions, WB-DWI scores were higher compared to FDG-PET-CT. DWI-MRI was of particular accurance in diagnosing diffuse disease (diffuse disease was observed in 37% of regions imaged on WB-DWI scans versus only 7% on FDG-PET-CT); both techniques were equally sensitive in the detection of focal lesions. [56] Preliminary reports suggest that DWI-MRI may be used for the better definition of response to therapy, but this has to be confirmed in larger studies and in comparison with PET-CT results [48, 57].

The dynamic contrast-enhanced MRI (DCE-MRI) is another MRI technique which evaluates the distribution of a contrast agent inside and outside the blood vessels. Information is assessed by computer-based analysis of repeated images over time. The analysis provides data for blood volume and vessel permeability for the assessment of microcirculation of a specific area [58, 59]. More importantly in MM patients, DCE-MRI-derived parameters correlated with marrow angiogenesis, microvessel density (MVD) [60], as well as in angiogenic response to therapy [61]. Regarding DCE-MRI sampling rate and model, there are two pharmacokinetic models (proposed by Brix and Tofts) that have been applied in the literature. However, a comparison of these models demonstrated that the Brix model is a little bit more robust [62]. Since DCE-MRI has not been established in clinical routine, no definite sequence can be recommended.

Positron emission tomography in combination with MRI (PET-MRI) represents a novel imaging modality in which the PET part detects active focal lesions, while the MRI part shows the location of the lesions and gives information on myeloma cell infiltration of the bone marrow. Especially in patients who reach a complete remission (CR), this technique might be able to localize residual sites of disease activity and therefore may help to guide treatment in the future [63]. In MM, there is only one prospective study, which compared PET-MRI with PET-CT in 30 myeloma patients with both techniques performed sequentially. There was high correlation between the two techniques, regarding number of active lesions and average SUV [64]. Further studies with PET-MRI will reveal if there is any value of this technique for MM patients.

MRI Patterns of Marrow Involvement. Five MRI patterns of bone marrow infiltration in myeloma have been reported: (1) normal appearance of bone marrow, (2) focal involvement (positive focal lesion is considered the lesion of a diameter of at least 5 mm), (3) homogeneous diffuse infiltration, (4) combined diffuse and focal infiltration, and (5) variegated or "salt-and-pepper" pattern with inhomogeneous bone marrow with interposition of fat islands [65, 66]. Low tumor burden is usually associated with a normal MRI pattern, but a high tumor burden is usually suspected when there is diffuse hypointense change on T1-weighted images, diffuse hyperintensity on T2-weighted images, and enhancement with gadolinium injection [67]. In several studies, the percentage of symptomatic patients with each of the abnormal MRI bone marrow patterns ranges from 18 to 50% for focal pattern, 25 to 43% for diffuse pattern, and 1 to 5% for variegated pattern [59]. The Durie-Salmon PLUS system uses the number of focal lesions (from focal or combined focal/diffuse patterns) for the staging of a myeloma patient and not the diffuse or "salt-and-pepper" patterns [68].

MRI Versus Conventional Radiography and Other Imaging Techniques for the Detection of Bone Involvement in Symptomatic Myeloma. MRI is more sensitive compared to WBXR for the detection of bone involvement in MM. In the largest series of patients published to date, MRI was compared to WBXR in 611 patients who received tandem autologous transplantation (ASCT). MRI and WBXR detected focal and osteolytic lesions in 74% and 56% of the imaged anatomic sites, respectively. Furthermore, 52% of 267 patients with normal WBXR had focal lesions on MRI. More precisely, MRI detected more focal lesions compared to lytic lesions in WBXR in the spine (78% vs. 16%; $p < 0.001$), the pelvis (64% vs. 28%; $p < 0.001$), and the sternum (24% vs. 3%; $p < 0.001$). WBXR had better performance than MRI in the ribs (10% vs. 43%; $p < 0.001$) and the long bones (37% vs. 48%; $p = 0.006$) and equal results in the skull and the shoulders [69]. Similar results had been previously reported in smaller studies, where MRI was superior to WBXR for the detection of focal vs. osteolytic lesions in the pelvis (75% vs. 46% of patients) and the spine (76% vs. 42%), especially in the lumbar spine [70–74]. A recent meta-analysis confirmed the superiority of MRI over WBXR regarding the detection of focal lesions and showed that MRI especially outscores WBXR in the axial skeleton but not in the ribs [75].

Although it is clear that MRI can detect bone marrow focal lesions long before the development of osteolytic lesions in the WBXR, other imaging techniques such as PET combined with computed tomography (PET-CT), CT, or WBCT detect more osteolytic lesions compared to WBXR [75]. Is there any evidence that MRI is superior to the other techniques in depicting bone involvement in myeloma? In a study with 41 newly diagnosed MM patients, WB-MRI was found superior to WBCT in detecting lesions in the skeleton [76]. In a prospective study, Zamagni et al. compared MRI of the spine and pelvis with WBXR and PET-CT in 46 MM patients at diagnosis. Although PET-CT was superior to WBXR in detecting lytic lesions in 46% of patients (19% had negative WBXR), it failed to reveal abnormal findings in 30% of patients who had abnormal MRI in the same areas, mainly of diffuse pattern. In that study, the combination of spine and pelvic MRI with PET-CT detected both medullary and extramedullary active myeloma sites in almost all patients (92%) [77]. Nevertheless, the Arkansas group was not able to confirm any superiority of MRI over PET-CT in the detection of more focal lesions in a large number of patients ($n = 303$) within the total therapy three protocols [78]. Still, in 188 patients who had at least one focal lesion in MRI, MRI was superior to PET-CT regarding the detection of higher number of focal lesions ($p = 0.032$). Furthermore, in this study, the presence of diffuse marrow pattern was not taken into consideration as an abnormal MRI finding [78]. Compared to sestamibitechnetium-99 m (MIBI) scan, WB-MRI detected more lesions in the vertebrae and the long bones, produced similar results in the skull, and was inferior in the ribs [79]. One important question in this point is the value of WB-MRI, which is not available everywhere, over the MRI of the spine and pelvis. In 100 patients with MM and MGUS who underwent WB-MRI, 10% presented with focal lesions merely in the extra-axial skeleton. These lesions would have been ignored if only MRI of the spine and pelvis had been performed [80].

Other advantages of MRI over WBXR and CT include the discrimination of myeloma from normal marrow [41, 81]; this finding can help in the differential diagnosis between myeloma and benign cause of a vertebral fracture. This is of extreme importance in cases of patients with a vertebral fracture and no other CRAB criteria and no lytic lesions. The MRI can also accurately illustrate the spinal cord and/or nerve root compression for surgical intervention or radiation therapy [29, 41]. Furthermore, the presence of soft tissue extension of MM and the presence of extramedullary plasmacytomas that are developed in approximately 10–20% of patients during the course of their disease can be precisely visualized by WB-MRI [82–85]. MRI can also help in the better evaluation of avascular necrosis of the femoral head [85] and the presence of soft tissue amyloid deposits [86]. Moreover, the tumor load can be assessed and monitored by MRI even in patients with nonsecretory and oligosecretory MM [87].

In conclusion, according to the latest IMWG guidelines, MRI is the gold standard imaging technique for the detection of bone marrow involvement in MM (grade A). MRI detects bone marrow involvement and not bone destruction. MRI of the spine and pelvis can detect approximately 90% of focal lesions in MM, and thus it can be used in cases where WB-MRI is not available (grade B). MRI is the procedure of choice to evaluate a painful lesion in myeloma patients, mainly in the axial skeleton, and to detect spinal cord compression (grade A). MRI is particularly useful in the evaluation of collapsed vertebrae, especially when myeloma is not active, where the possibility of osteoporotic fracture is high (grade B) [88].

Prognostic Value of MRI. The prognostic significance of MRI findings in symptomatic myeloma has been evaluated. The largest study in the literature included 611 patients who received tandem ASCT-based protocols. Focal lesions detected by spinal MRI and not seen on WBXR independently correlated with overall survival (OS). Resolution of the focal lesions on MRI posttreatment occurred in 60% of the patients who had superior survival. At disease progression after complete response (CR), MRI revealed new focal lesions in 26% of patients, enlargement of previous focal lesions in 28% of patients, and both features in 15% of patients [69]. In a more recent analysis of the same group on 429 patients, patients who had >7 focal lesions in MRI ($n = 147$) had a 73% probability of 3-year OS vs. 86% for those who had 0–7 focal lesions ($n = 235$) and 81% for those who had diffuse pattern of marrow infiltration ($n = 47$; $p = 0.04$). PET-CT and WBXR also produced similar results in the univariate analysis. In the multivariate analysis, from the imaging variables, only the presence of >2 osteolytic lesions in WBXR at diagnosis and the presence of >3 focal lesions in the PET-CT, 7 days post-ASCT had independent prognostic value for inferior OS ($p = 0.01$ and 0.03, respectively). However, we have to mention the high percentage of patients (232/429, 54%) who had no detectable osteolytic lesions by WBXR and the absence of evaluation of diffuse MRI pattern in this study [89].

The MRI pattern of marrow infiltration has also reported to have prognostic significance in newly diagnosed patients with symptomatic disease [67, 90, 91]. In the conventional chemotherapy (CC) era, Moulopoulos et al. published that the median OS of newly diagnosed MM patients was 24 months if they had diffuse MRI pattern versus 51, 52, and 56 months for those with focal, variegated, and normal patterns, respectively, ($p = 0.001$) [67]. This is possibly because diffuse MRI marrow pattern correlates with increased angiogenesis and advanced disease features [92, 93]. The same group also reported the prognostic value of MRI patterns in 228 symptomatic MM patients who received upfront regimens based on novel agents. Patients with diffuse pattern had inferior survival compared to patients with other MRI patterns; moreover, the combination of diffuse MRI pattern, ISS-3 stage, and high risk cytogenetics could identify a group of patients with very poor survival: median of 21 months and a probability of 3-year OS of only 35% [91]. Another study in 126 patients with newly diagnosed symptomatic myeloma who underwent an ASCT showed that the diffuse and the variegated MRI patterns had an independent predictive value for disease progression (HR: 1.922; $p = 0.008$) [93]. Finally, in patients with progressive or relapsed MM, an increased signal of DCE-MRI offered shorter PFS, possibly due to its association with higher MVD [58].

MRI and Response to Antimyeloma Therapy. An interesting finding is that a change in MRI pattern correlates with response to therapy. Moulopoulos et al. firstly reported in the era of CC that CR is characterized by complete resolution of the preceding marrow abnormality, while partial response (PR) is characterized by changeover of diffuse pattern to variegated or focal patterns [94]. In a retrospective study that was conducted in the era of novel agents, response to treatment was compared with changes in infiltration patterns of WB-MRI before and after ASCT ($n = 100$). There was a strong correlation between response to antimyeloma therapies and changes in both diffuse ($p = 0.004$) and focal ($p = 0.01$) MRI patterns. Furthermore, the number of focal lesions at second MRI was of prognostic significance for OS ($p = 0.001$) [95]. Another study in 33 patients who underwent an ASCT showed that WB-MRI data demonstrated progressive disease in ten patients (30%) and response to high-dose therapy in 23 (70%). Eight (80%) of the ten patients with progressive disease revealed intramedullary lesions, and two patients (20%) had intra- and extramedullary lesions. WB-MRI had a sensitivity of 64%, specificity of 86%, positive predictive value of 70%, negative predictive value of

83%, and accuracy of 79% for detection of remission [96]. This study supports that one of the disadvantages of MRI is that it often provides false-positive results because of persistent nonviable lesions. Thus, PET-CT might be more suitable than MRI for determination of remission status [97]. Indeed in a large study of 191 patients, PET-CT revealed faster change of imaging findings than MRI in patients who responded to therapy [98]. It seems that the PET-CT normalization after treatment can offer more information compared to MRI for the better definition of CR [99].

To improve the results of MRI for the most accurate detection of remission, the DW-MRI has been recently used. In a first preliminary report, ADC values in active myeloma were significantly higher than marrow in remission [50]. Furthermore, the mean ADC increased in 95% of responding patients and decreased in all ($n = 5$) nonresponders ($p = 0.002$). An increase of ADC by 3.3% was associated with response, having a sensitivity of 90% and specificity of 100%. Furthermore, there was a negative correlation between changes of ADC and changes of biochemical markers of response ($r = -0.614$; $p = 0.001$) [100]. Large prospective clinical studies are definitely justified by these results.

The Value of MRI in the Definition of Smoldering/Asymptomatic Myeloma. The presence of lytic lesions by WBXR is included in the definition of symptomatic myeloma, based on studies showing that patients with at least one lytic lesion in WBXR have a median time to progression (TTP) of 10 months [101]. However, in patients with no osteolytic lesions in WBXR, the MRI reveals abnormal marrow appearance in 20–50% of them [66, 67, 102–104]; these patients are at higher risk for progression. Moulopoulos et al. reported that patients with SMM and abnormal MRI studies required therapy after a median of 16 months vs. 43 months for those with normal MRI ($p < 0.01$) [102]. Hillengass and colleagues evaluated WB-MRI in 149 SMM patients. Focal lesions were detected in 42 (28%) patients, while >1 focal lesion was present in 23 patients (15%) who had high risk of progression (HR = 4.05, $p < 0.001$). The median TTP was 13 months, and the progression rate at 2 years was 70%. On multivariate analysis, presence of >1 focal lesion remained a significant predictor of progression after adjusting for other risk factors including bone marrow plasmacytosis, serum and urine M-protein levels, and suppression of uninvolved immunoglobulins. In the same study, the diffuse marrow infiltration on MRI was also associated with increased risk for progression (HR = 3.5, $p < 0.001$) [103]. Kastritis and colleagues also showed in 98 SMM patients that abnormal marrow pattern in the MRI of the spine, which was present in 21% of patients, was associated with high risk of progression with a median TTP to symptomatic myeloma of 15 months ($p = 0.001$) [104].

An important issue is whether patients who have two or more small focal lesions (<5 mm) should be considered as patients with symptomatic myeloma and how to manage them. The Heidelberg group analyzed very recently data of 63 SMM patients who had at least two WB-MRIs performed for follow-up before progression into symptomatic disease. The definition of radiological progression according to MRI findings included one of the following: (1) development of a new focal lesion, (2) increase of the diameter of an existing focal lesion, and (3) detection of novel or progressive diffuse MRI pattern. The second MRI was performed 3–6 months after the performance of the first MRI. Evaluation of response according to IMWG criteria was also performed. Progressive disease according to MRI was observed in approximately 50% of patients, while 40% of patients developed symptomatic MM based on the CRAB criteria. In the multivariate analysis, MRI-PD was an independent prognostic factor for progression. Patients with stable MRI findings had no higher risk of progression, even when focal lesions were present at the initial MRI [105]. Prospective clinical trials should be conducted to confirm the above findings.

MRI Findings in Monoclonal Gammopathy of Undetermined Significance (MGUS). MGUS by definition is characterized by the absence of osteolytic lesions. However, MGUS patients have higher incidence of osteoporosis and vertebral fractures compared to normal population [106, 107]. In a small study which included 37 patients with MGUS or SMM, MRI abnormalities were detected in 20% of them. These patients had a higher time to progression (TTP) to symptomatic myeloma compared to patients with a normal MRI who did not progress after a median follow-up of 30 months [108]. A prospective study in 331 patients with MGUS or SMM revealed that the detection of multiple (>1) focal lesions by MRI conferred an increased risk of progression [109]. In another large study, which included only MGUS patients ($n = 137$) who underwent a WB-MRI at diagnosis, a focal infiltration pattern was detected in 23% of them. Independent prognostic factors for progression to symptomatic myeloma included the presence and number of focal lesions and the value of M-protein [110].

MRI and Solitary Plasmacytoma of the Bone (SPB). The diagnosis of SBP includes the presence of a solitary bone lesion, with a confirmed infiltration by plasma cells in the biopsy of the lesion, absence of clonal plasma cells in the trephine bone marrow biopsy, and no CRAB criteria. Although definitive radiotherapy usually eradicates the local disease, the majority of patients will develop MM because of the growth of previously occult lesions which have not been detected by WBXR [83]. Moulopoulos et al. published that spinal MRI revealed additional focal lesions in 4/12 SBP patients. After treatment with radiotherapy to the painful lesion, three patients developed systemic disease within 18 months from diagnosis [82]. Furthermore, Liebross et al. observed that among SBP patients with spinal disease, 7/8 staged by WBXR alone developed MM compared to only 1/7 patients who also had spinal MRI [111].

8.7 PET-CT

PET-CT Detection of Bone Involvement in Myeloma. FDG-PET-CT is a functional imaging method, which combines demonstration of hypermetabolic activity in intramedullary and extramedullary sites (PET) with evidence of osteolysis (CT). Several studies have shown that PET-CT is more sensitive compared to WBXR for the detection of osteolytic lesions in MM [77, 112–114]. This has been confirmed by the largest meta-analysis in the field [75]. The higher detection rate of PET-CT over WBXR for the presence of osteolytic lesions is especially important for patients with SMM. In one study with 120 patients with SMM based on the previous IMWG criteria [77], 16% of patients with normal WBXR had positive PET-CT results. The median time to progression (TTP) for PET-CT-positive patients was 1.1 years vs. 4.5 for patients with negative PET-CT, while the probability of progression at 2 years for PET-CT-positive patients was 58% [115]. The largest study in the field involved 188 with suspected SMM examined with PET-CT. PET-CT was positive in 39% of patients. The probability of progression to symptomatic MM within 2 years was 75% for patients with a positive PET-CT under observation versus only 30% for patients with a negative PET-CT. This probability was higher if hypermetabolic activity was combined with underlying osteolysis (2-year progression rate: 87%). The median TTP was 21 months vs. 60 months for PET-CT-positive and PET-CT-negative patients, respectively [116]. The results of these two studies support the integration of changes in imaging requirements in the new IMWG diagnostic criteria for MM; detection of osteolytic lesions by PET-CT is a criterion for symptomatic MM [14].

Compared to MRI, as mentioned previously, PET-CT performs equally well in detecting focal lesions, but MRI is better in detecting diffuse disease [76, 77, 114].

Value of PET-CT for Better Definition of Complete Response to Antimyeloma Therapy. Data obtained from PET-CT in 40 MM patients, including average SUV and FDG kinetic parameters K1, influx, and fractal dimension, correlated significantly with percentage of bone marrow infiltration on trephine biopsies (PC %) [117]. Furthermore, PET-CT efficiently detected extramedullary disease in patients both at diagnosis and at relapse [118]. Consequently, PET-CT was tested for better definition of CR in 282 MM patients. It was performed at diagnosis and every 12–18 months afterward. At diagnosis, 42% of MM patients had >3 focal lesions; in 50% of these patients SUV max was >4.2. After treatment, PET-CT was negative in 70% of patients, while 53% of patients achieved CR according to IMWG criteria. Approximately 30% of patients at CR had positive PET-CT. More importantly, PET-CT negativity was an independent predictor for prolonged PFS and OS in CR patients; median PFS was 50 months for PET-CT-positive and 90 months for PET-CT-negative CR patients [119]. PET-CT, therefore, provides more accurate definition of CR, and it has been suggested that it should be incorporated to CR criteria [120].

Prognostic Significance of PET-CT. Several studies have confirmed the value of PET-CT as an independent factor for survival in MM patients both at diagnosis and posttreatment [99, 121–125]. In 192 newly diagnosed patients who underwent ASCT, the presence of extramedullary disease and SUVmax >4.2 on PET-CT performed at diagnosis, as well as the persistence of FDG uptake post-ASCT were independent variables, adversely affecting PFS [121]. In the largest study in the field, 429 patients who were treated with total therapy protocols in Arkansas were evaluated with both MRI and PET-CT at diagnosis and 7 days post-ASCT. From the imaging variables, in the multivariate analysis, only the detection of >2 osteolytic lesions by WBXR at diagnosis and the detection of >3 focal lesions by PET-CT, 7 days post-ASCT, were independent prognostic factors for inferior

OS. Limitation of this study was the exclusion of diffuse MRI pattern from the analysis [89]. Despite this limitation, studies reported to-date support the role of PET-CT after therapy, deeming it the best imaging technique for the follow-up of myeloma patients. Indeed, in a recent study which has been reported only in an abstract form, 134 patients who were eligible for treatment with ASCT were randomized to receive 8 cycles of bortezomib-lenalidomide-dexamethasone (VRD) followed by 1-year maintenance with lenalidomide or 3 cycles of VRD followed by ASCT plus 2 cycles of VRD consolidation and 1-year lenalidomide maintenance. PET-CT and WB-MRI were performed after induction and before maintenance. Both techniques were positive at diagnosis in more than 90% of patients. After induction therapy and before maintenance, more patients continued to have positive MRI than PET-CT (93% vs. 55%, and 83% vs. 21%, respectively), possibly due to earlier reduction of activity of PET-CT lesions. Both after induction and before maintenance, normalization of PET-CT and not of MRI could predict for PFS, while only normalization of PET-CT before maintenance could predict for OS (30-month OS rate: 70% in PET-CT-positive patients vs. 94.6% in patients with negative PET-CT negative; $p = 0.01$) [126].

At this point, it is crucial to mention that one of the major limitations of PET-CT is the lack of standardization and the controversies regarding SUV level of positivity. Recently, an Italian panel of experts introduced novel criteria for the interpretation of PET-CT images [127]. Large, multicenter, studies with prospective evaluation of these new criteria will reveal their clinical impact.

Other PET-CT Indications and Limitations. PET-CT may be used for the work-up of patients with SBP at diagnosis [128]. However, it is not clear whether PET-CT or MRI is more suitable in this setting since restaging PET-CT after radiotherapy has a number of false-positive findings [129]. PET-CT also has a role in patients with nonsecretory or oligo-secretory myeloma for the detection of active lesions in the body [130]. Major limitations of PET-CT include high cost, lack of availability in many centers and countries, and false-positive results due to inflammation of other underlying pathology.

8.8 Management of Multiple Myeloma Bone Disease

Bisphosphonates (BPs) are the mainstay in the management of MM bone disease. They are artificial analogues of pyrophosphates. In comparison with natural pyrophosphates, bisphosphonates are resistant to phosphatase-induced hydrolysis [131]. Bisphosphonates cause osteoclast suppression. They bind to calcium containing molecules such as hydroxyapatite [132]. Osteoclast-induced bone resorption causes exposure of hydroxyapatite. Bisphosphonates bind to the exposed molecules of hydroxyapatite. This fact leads to increased concentration of bisphosphonates within the lytic lesions [132–134]. There are two main groups of bisphosphonates, each with a differently proposed mechanism of action [132]. Non-nitrogen-containing bisphosphonates induce osteoclast apoptosis via their cytotoxic ATP analogues. On the other hand, nitrogen-containing bisphosphonates downregulate osteoclast activity by inhibiting the HMG-CoA reductase pathway. Etidronate and clodronate (CLO) are non-nitrogen-containing bisphosphonates. Zoledronic acid (ZOL), ibandronate, pamidronate (PAM), and risedronate are nitrogen-containing bisphosphonates. All bisphosphonates have similar physicochemical properties; however, their anti-resorbing activity is different. Their activity is drastically increased when an amino group is entered into the aliphatic carbon chain. Thus, pamidronate is 100- and 700-fold more potent than etidronate, both in vitro and in vivo, while zoledronic acid and ibandronate show 10,000- to 100,000-fold greater potency than etidronate [135]. Bisphosphonates also appear to affect the microenvironment in which tumor cells grow and may have direct antitumor activity [136–141]. Possible mechanisms include the reduction of IL-6 secretion by bone marrow stromal cells or the expansion of gamma/delta T cells with possible anti-MM activity. The aim of bisphosphonates use is the reduction of SREs in patients with myeloma bone disease [23].

According to the latest IMWG guidelines, bisphosphonates should be initiated in MM patients, with (grade A) or without (grade B) detectable osteolytic bone lesions in conventional radiography, who are receiving antimyeloma therapy, as well as patients with osteoporosis (grade A) or osteopenia (grade C) due to myeloma. The beneficial effect of zoledronic acid in patients without detectable bone disease by MRI or PET-CT is not known. Oral clodronate, intravenous pamidronate, and intravenous zoledronic acid have been licensed for the management of myeloma bone disease. Etidronate and ibandronate were found to be ineffective for the treatment of bone disease in myeloma patients [142, 143]. Several studies have evaluated the effects of bisphosphonates (BPs) on SREs and bone pain in patients with MM [144].

8.8.1 Etidronate

Etidronate was found to be ineffective in two placebo-controlled studies in myeloma patients [142, 145].

8.8.2 Ibandronate

Ibandronate is ineffective in reducing SREs or improving bone pain in patients with MM [143].

8.8.3 Clodronate

The oral BP, clodronate, reduced the proportion of patients with MM who experienced progression of osteolytic lesions by 50% compared with placebo (24% vs. 12%; $P = 0.026$) 24 and reduced the time to first and the rate of nonvertebral fracture (6.8% vs. 13.2% for placebo; $P = 0.04$) in patients with newly diagnosed MM [13]. Two major, placebo-controlled, randomized trials have been performed in

MM. Lahtinen et al. reported reduction of the development of new osteolytic lesions by 50% in myeloma patients who received oral CLO for 2 years that was independent of the presence of lytic lesions at baseline [146]. In the other study, although there was no difference in overall survival (OS) between CLO and placebo patients, patients who received CLO and did not have vertebral fractures at baseline appeared to have a survival advantage (59 vs. 37 months). Both vertebral and nonvertebral fractures as well as the time to first nonvertebral fracture and severe hypercalcemia were reduced in the CLO group after 1 year of follow-up, and at 2 years, the patients who received CLO had better performance status and less myeloma-related pain than patients treated with placebo [147].

8.8.4 Pamidronate

PAM is an aminobisphosphonate, which has been administered either orally or intravenously. In one trial, patients with advanced disease and at least one lytic lesion were randomized to placebo or intravenous PAM [148]. Administration of PAM resulted in a significant reduction in skeletal-related events (SREs; 24%) vs. placebo (41%; $p < 0.001$). Patients receiving PAM also experienced reduced bone pain and no deterioration in quality of life (QoL) during the 2-year study. By contrast, administration of oral PAM failed to reduce SREs relative to placebo [149]. However, patients treated with oral PAM experienced fewer episodes of severe pain. The overall negative result of this study was attributed to the low absorption of orally administered BPs [149]. A recent study for patients with newly diagnosed MM demonstrated that PAM 30 mg monthly had comparable time with SREs and SRE-free survival time as compared with PAM 90 mg monthly. After a minimum of 3 years, patients receiving PAM 30 mg showed a trend toward lower risks of osteonecrosis of the jaw (ONJ) and nephrotoxicity compared with the higher dose. However, the study was not powered to show SRE differences between the two PAM dosages but only to show QoL differences [150].

8.8.5 Zoledronic Acid (ZOL)

In a non-inferiority randomized phase II trial published by Berenson et al., escalating doses of ZOL were tested in comparison with 90 mg of PAM, in 280 patients, 108 of them affected by MM (the other had metastatic breast cancer to bone). Both ZOL (at doses of 2 and 4 mg) and PAM significantly reduced SREs in contrast to 0.4 mg ZOL [151]. This phase II trial failed to show any superiority of ZOL compared with PAM in terms of SREs, but it was not powered to show differences between the groups.

Bisphosphonates Head to Head. There are only two large randomized studies comparing two different BPs. A phase III, randomized, double-blind study was performed to compare the effects of zoledronic acid with pamidronate for patients with myeloma and lytic bone disease or with metastatic breast cancer to bone [152, 153].

In the myeloma cohort, there was no difference between the two treatment arms regarding incidence and time to first SRE. However, N-terminal cross-linking telopeptide of collagen type I (NTX) levels, a sensitive marker of bone resorption, normalized more often in the zoledronic acid arm compared with pamidronate-treated patients. More recently, the Medical Research Council (MRC) of the UK compared zoledronic acid (4 mg intravenous every 3–4 weeks or at doses according to creatinine clearance [CrCl] rates) and oral clodronate (1600 mg orally daily) for patients with newly diagnosed, symptomatic MM, who were treated with antimyeloma therapy (n = 1960 evaluable for efficacy). Zoledronic acid reduced the incidence of SREs both in myeloma patients with or without bone lesions as assessed using conventional radiography, compared with clodronate [154, 155]. After a median follow-up of 3.7 years, 35% of patients receiving clodronate had experienced SREs vs. 27% of patients receiving zoledronic acid (p = 0.004). More importantly, zoledronic acid reduced mortality and extended median survival. Further, subset analysis showed this treatment extended survival by 10 months over clodronate for patients with osteolytic disease at diagnosis, whereas myeloma patients without bone disease at diagnosis as assessed using conventional radiography had no survival advantage with zoleronic acid [155]. These results confirm preclinical studies suggesting indirect and direct antimyeloma effects of zoledronic acid [156]. Possible mechanisms for the antimyeloma effects of zoledronic acid include direct cytotoxic effect on the tumor cells, the reduction of IL-6 secretion by bone marrow stromal cells, the expansion of gamma/delta T cells with possible anti-MM activity, antiangiogenic effects, and inhibitory effects in the adhesion molecules. In specific subsets of patients, other BPs have also been associated with improved survival: patients receiving second-line antimyeloma chemotherapy and treated with pamidronate experienced a borderline improvement in OS over placebo [148], whereas clodronate had an OS advantage in patients without vertebral fractures at presentation relative to placebo [147]. Nevertheless, a Cochrane database meta-analysis showed that zoledronic acid was the only BP associated with superior OS compared with placebo (hazard ratio, 0.61; 95% CI, 0.28–0.98), but not compared with other BPs [157].

Patients with Asymptomatic Myeloma (AMM). Intravenous PAM (60–90 mg monthly for 12 months) in patients with AMM reduced bone involvement at progression but did not decrease the risk and increase the time to progression [158]. Similarly, intravenous ZOL (4 mg monthly for 12 months) reduced the SRE risk at progression but did not influence the risk of progression of AMM patients [159].

Several studies have reported the value of MRI (presence of >1 focal lesion and presence of diffuse pattern of marrow infiltration) in detecting patients with AMM at high risk for progression [102, 103]. Since there is no data supporting PFS advantage with bisphosphonates in AMM, bisphosphonates should not be recommended except for a clinical trial of high-risk patients.

Patients with MGUS. MGUS patients are at high risk for developing osteoporosis and pathological fractures [160, 161]. Three doses of ZOL (4 mg intravenously every 6 months) increased bone mineral density (BMD) by 15% in the lumbar spine and by 6% in the femoral neck in MGUS patients with osteopenia or osteoporosis

[162]. Oral alendronate (70 mg/weekly) also increased BMD of the lumbar spine and total femur by 6.1% and 1.5%, respectively, in 50 MGUS patients with vertebral fractures and/or osteoporosis [163].

Patients with Solitary Plasmacytoma (SPB). Patients with solitary plasmacytoma and no evidence of MM do not require therapy with bisphosphonates. However, these patients should have a whole-body MRI since in a study of 17 patients diagnosed with a solitary plasmacytoma, all showed additional focal lesions or a diffuse infiltration on MRI, leading to a classification as stage I MM (76%), stage II MM (12%), or stage III MM (12%) using the Durie-Salmon PLUS system [164].

Route of Administration. Strict adherence to dosing recommendations is required for bisphosphonate therapy to effectively reduce and delay SREs in patients with MM. Each patient prescribed bisphosphonate therapy should be instructed about the crucial importance of adherence to the dosing regimen. Although a few randomized, placebo-controlled clinical studies suggest that long-term compliance with oral bisphosphonates such as CLO is satisfactory in MM patients [13, 146], compliance with oral bisphosphonate therapy is generally suboptimal [165]. Further, the MRC-IX data strongly support the use of intravenous ZOL over CLO in all outcomes measured, including reduction of SREs and improvement in OS [154, 155, 166]. According to the latest IMWG guidelines, intravenous administration of BPs is the preferred choice (grade A). However, oral administration remains an option for patients who cannot receive regular hospital care or in-home nursing visits (grade D) [144].

Treatment Duration. Intravenous bisphosphonates should be administered at 3- to 4-week intervals to all patients with active MM (grade A). ZOL improves OS and reduces SREs over CLO in patients who received treatment for more than 2 years; thus, it should be given until disease progression in patients not in complete remission (CR) or a very good partial remission (VGPR) and further continued at relapse (grade B). There is not similar evidence for PAM. PAM may be continued in patients with active disease at the physician's discretion (grade D), and PAM therapy should be resumed after disease relapse (grade D). For patients in CR/VGPR, the optimal treatment duration of BPs is not clear. According to the IMWG, BPs should be given for at least 12 months and up to 24 months and then at the physician's discretion (grade D; panel consensus).

According to the latest IMWG guidelines and due to higher reported rates of ONJ with extended duration of therapy, ZOL or PAM should be discontinued after 1–2 years in patients who have achieved CR or VGPR (grade D; panel consensus) [144].

8.8.6 Adverse Events

Even though bisphosphonate therapy is well tolerated in patients with MM, clinicians should be alert for symptoms and signs suggesting adverse events (AEs), and patients and healthcare professionals should be instructed on how to prevent and recognize AEs. Potential AEs associated with bisphosphonate administration include hypocalcemia and hypophosphatemia, gastrointestinal events after oral administration, inflammatory reactions at the injection site, and acute-phase reactions after IV administration of aminobisphosphonates. Renal impairment and ONJ represent infrequent but potentially serious AEs with bisphosphonate use.

Hypocalcemia. Hypocalcemia is usually relatively mild and asymptomatic with bisphosphonate use in most MM patients. The incidence of symptomatic hypocalcemia is much lower in MM patients compared to patients with solid tumors. Although severe hypocalcemia has been observed in some patients [167], it is usually preventable via the administration of oral calcium and vitamin D3. Patients should routinely receive calcium (600 mg/day) and vitamin D3 (400 IU/day) supplementation since 60% of MM patients have vitamin D deficiency or insufficiency [168, 169]. In vitamin D-deficient patients, there is an increase in bone remodeling. This fact shows that MM patients should be calcium and vitamin D sufficient [170]. Calcium supplementation should be used with caution in patients with renal insufficiency.

Renal Impairment. Bisphosphonate infusions are associated with both dose- and infusion rate-dependent effects on renal function. The potential for renal damage is dependent on the concentration of bisphosphonate in the bloodstream, and the highest risk is observed after administration of high dosages or rapid infusion. Both ZOL and PAM have been associated with acute renal damage or increases in serum creatinine [152, 171]. Patients should be closely monitored for compromised renal function by measuring CrCl before administration of each IV bisphosphonate infusion. Current guideline recommendations [144] state that the dosages of zoledronic acid and clodronate, when administered intravenously, should be reduced for patients who have preexisting renal impairment (CrCl 30–60 mL/min), but there are no clinical studies demonstrating the efficacy of this approach. For patients with CrCl between 30–60 mL/min, zoledronic acid dose should be adjusted. Zoledronic acid has not been studied for patients presented with severe renal impairment (CrCl <30 mL/min), and it is not recommended for patients with severe renal impairment (CrCl <30 mL/min). We suggest that pamidronate may be given at a dose of 90 mg infused over 4–6 h for myeloma patients with osteolytic disease and renal insufficiency. Furthermore, serum creatinine and CrCl should be measured before each infusion of pamidronate or zoledronic acid, while BPs should not be administered in short infusion times (<2 h for pamidronate and less than 15 min for zoledronic acid). Bisphosphonate therapy can be resumed, after withholding zoledronic acid or pamidronate for patients who develop renal deterioration during therapy, when serum creatinine returns to within 10% of baseline [144].

Osteonecrosis of the Jaw. It is an uncommon complication of intravenous bisphosphonates. It is potentially serious, and its main characteristic is the presence of exposed bone in the mouth. Incidence may vary from 2 to 10% [172, 173]. Longer exposure increases the cumulative incidence of ONJ. One of the main risk factors for the development of ONJ is the invasive dental procedures [172]. Other risk factors include poor oral hygiene, age, and duration of myeloma. Zoledronic acid was associated with a higher incidence of ONJ in retrospective evaluations [174]. In approximately one half of patients, ONJ lesions will heal [175], but approximately one half of patients who restart bisphosphonate therapy after having stopped it will develop recurrence of ONJ. According to recent IMWG guidelines [176], preventive strategies should be adopted to avoid ONJ. A dental examination is necessary before beginning of the bisphosphonate's course. Patients should also be alerted regarding dental hygiene (grade C; panel consensus). All existing dental condition should be treated before initiation of bisphosphonate therapy (grade C; panel consensus). After bisphosphonate treatment initiation, unnecessary invasive dental procedures should be avoided, and dental health status should be monitored on annual basis (grade C). Patients' dental health status should be monitored by a physician and a dentist (grade D; panel consensus). Dental problems should be managed conservatively if possible (grade C). If invasive dental procedures are necessary, there should be temporary suspension of bisphosphonate treatment (grade D). The panel consensus suggests the interruption of bisphosphonates before and after dental procedures for a total of 180 days (90 days before and 90 days after procedures such as tooth extraction, dental implants, and surgery to the jaw). Bisphosphonates do not need to be discontinued for routine dental procedures including root canal. Initial treatment of ONJ should include discontinuation of bisphosphonates until healing occurs (grade C). The physician should consider the advantages and disadvantages of continued treatment with bisphosphonates, especially in the relapsed/refractory MM setting (grade D). Preventive measures during bisphosphonate treatment have the potential to reduce the incidence of ONJ about 75% [177]. Prophylactic antibiotic treatment may prevent ONJ occurrence after dental procedures [178]. Management of patients depends on ONJ stage. Stage I (asymptomatic exposed bone, no soft tissue infection) can be managed conservatively with oral antimicrobial rinses. Stage II (exposed bone and associated pain/swelling and/or soft tissue infection) requires culture-directed long-term and maintenance antimicrobial therapy, analgesic management, and, occasionally, minor bony debridement. Stage III disease (pathological fracture and exposed bone or soft tissue infection not manageable with antibiotics) requires surgical resection in order to reduce the volume of necrotic bone in addition to the measures described in stage II [179]. When ONJ occurs, initial therapy should include discontinuation of bisphosphonates until healing occurs [132]. The administration of medical ozone (O3) as an oil suspension directly to the ONJ lesions that are below ≤2.5 cm may be another possible therapeutic strategy for those patients who fail to respond to conservative treatment. In such patients, there are reports suggesting that ONJ lesions resolved with complete reconstitution of oral and jaw tissue, with 3–10 applications [180, 181]. In addition, treatment with hyperbaric oxygen has been reported to be helpful.

8.9 Future Treatment Options

8.9.1 RANKL/RANK Pathway Regulators: Targeting the Osteoclast

RANKL Antagonists. Preclinical models of MM demonstrated that RANKL inhibition can prevent bone destruction from MM. RANKL inhibition with recombinant RANK-Fc protein not only reduced MM-induced osteolysis but also caused a marked decline in tumor burden [182, 183]. Similar results were obtained using recombinant OPG for the treatment of MM-bearing animals [184]. These data gave the rationale for using RANKL inhibition in the clinical setting.

Denosumab, a fully human monoclonal antibody, has showed high affinity and specificity in binding RANKL and inhibits RANKL-RANK interaction, mimicking the endogenous effects of OPG. In knock-in mice with chimeric (murine/human) RANKL expression, denosumab showed inhibition of bone resorption [185].

In a phase I trial, 54 patients with breast cancer ($n = 29$) or MM ($n = 25$) with radiologically confirmed bone lesions received a single dose of either denosumab or pamidronate. Denosumab decreased bone resorption within 24 h of administration, as reflected by levels of urinary and serum NTX. That was similar in magnitude but more sustained than with intravenous pamidronate [186]. These results were confirmed in another phase I trial, in which denosumab was given at multiple doses [187].

In a phase II trial, the ability of denosumab (120 mg given monthly as a subcutaneous injection) to affect bone resorption markers and monoclonal protein levels in MM patients who relapsed after response to prior therapy and in patients with response to most recent therapy and who had stable disease for at least 3 months was evaluated. No patients experienced complete or partial response ($\geq 50\%$ reduction in M-protein), but seven patients had maximum reduction of $\geq 25\%$ in serum M-protein. Bone resorption markers were reduced by more than 50% with denosumab [188].

In another phase II trial, Fizazi et al. evaluated the effect of denosumab in patients with bone metastases and elevated urinary NTX levels despite ongoing intravenous bisphosphonate therapy. Patients were stratified by tumor type (total 111 patients: 9 patients with multiple myeloma, 50 patients with prostate cancer, 46 patients with breast cancer, and 6 patients with another solid tumor) and screening NTX levels and randomly assigned to receive subcutaneous denosumab 180 mg every four or every 12 weeks or continue intravenous bisphosphonates every 4 weeks. Denosumab normalized urinary NTX levels more frequently than the continuation of intravenous bisphosphonate (64% vs. 37%, respectively, $p = 0.01$), while fewer patients receiving denosumab experienced on-study SREs than those receiving intravenous bisphosphonate (8% vs. 17%) [189]. This study showed that denosumab inhibits bone resorption and prevents SREs even in patients who are refractory to bisphosphonate therapy.

A meta-analysis of major phase 3 studies comparing denosumab vs. zoledronic acid including mainly patients with solid tumors showed that denosumab was superior in terms of delaying the time to first on-study SRE by 8 months and reducing the risk of the first SRE by 17%. No difference between the two drugs was reported regarding disease progression and overall survival. Hypocalcaemia was more common in denosumab arm, while ONJ was similar with the two drugs [190].

Denosumab appears to have little toxicity, mainly asthenia, and multiple phase III trials of denosumab in patients with bone metastasis are ongoing. However, it is crucial to mention that RANKL is involved in dendritic cell survival and that the anti-RANKL strategy may have an effect on the immune system and a possible increase in infection rate, especially in cancer patients who have already had severe immunodeficiency. For MM patients, while denosumab was comparable to zoledronic acid with respect to the occurrence of SREs, inferior survival occurred in denosumab compared to zoledronic acid-treated patients, but this was a subset analysis from a large phase III trial that involved mostly solid tumor patients with metastatic bone disease [191]. Interpretation is limited based on the small numbers of MM patients who were enrolled on the trial and imbalance in baseline disease characteristics.

To address this survival discrepancy in the phase 3 RCT, a confirmatory phase 3 trial that included 1718 newly diagnosed myeloma patients, randomized to denosumab (758 patients) and zoledronic acid (758 patients), stratified by type of first-line therapy and previous SRE, was recently reported at the IMW 2017 [Raje et al. OP-46]. Primary endpoint was non-inferiority of denosumab (vs ZA) for time to first SRE while on study. Several secondary endpoints were evaluated including the superiority of denosumab and overall survival (OS). At a median follow-up of 17.4 months, median time to first on-study SRE was similar between both groups (23 months). 43.8% pts. on denosumab and 44.6% on ZA had a first on-study SRE ($P = 0.01$), confirming the non-inferiority of denosumab to ZA in delaying time to first on-study SRE (HR = 0.98[0.85,1.14]). More interestingly, a pre-specified exploratory endpoint, the PFS favored the denosumab arm (HR = 0.82[0.68,0.99]), $P = 0.036$. Denosumab met the primary endpoint of the study demonstrating the non-inferiority to ZA in delaying time to first SRE. The safety profile of denosumab is established. Though the lack of OS difference suggests a shorter follow-up of the study, it is reassuring to know that the inferiority in survival from earlier RCT was not demonstrated and will need further follow-up.

8.9.2   Activin-A Inhibitors

Sotatercept (ACE-011) is a fusion protein of the extracellular domain of the high-affinity activin receptor IIA (ActRIIA) and human immunoglobulin G (IgG) Fc domain with potent inhibitory effect on activin, enhancing the deposition of new bone tissue and preventing bone loss. In the preclinical setting, RAP-011, a murine counterpart of sotatercept, prevented the formation of osteolytic lesions in a murine MM model by stimulating bone formation through osteoblasts, while having no effect on osteoclast activity [192].

In a phase 1 study, in healthy postmenopausal volunteers, single-dose sotatercept was associated with increased serum levels of the bone formation marker bone-specific alkaline phosphatase (bALP) and decreased bone resorption markers CTX and tartrate-resistant acid phosphatase isoform 5b (TRACP-5b), reflecting a decrease in bone resorption and an increase in bone formation [193]. No safety concerns were noted in this study.

In a multicenter phase 2 trial, patients with osteolytic bone lesions due to MM were randomized to receive either four 28-day cycles of sotatercept or placebo as subcutaneous injection with concomitant anticancer therapy consisting of oral melphalan, prednisolone, and thalidomide (MPT). Sotatercept treatment demonstrated clinically significant increases in biomarkers of bone formation, decreases in bone pain, and antitumor activity as well as increase in hemoglobin levels [192], but further research is needed to support these findings. Moreover, increased activin-A secretion was induced by lenalidomide and was canceled by the addition of an activin-A-neutralizing antibody. This effectively restored osteoblast function and subsequently inhibited myeloma-related osteolysis without abrogating the cytotoxic effects of lenalidomide on malignant cells [194] and thus supporting the combination of lenalidomide with an anti-activin-A molecule.

8.10 Future Agents Targeting the Osteoclast

The pathophysiology of myeloma bone disease is complex. Interactions between myeloma cells, stromal cells, osteoclasts, and osteoblasts create vicious cycles that lead to the development of osteolytic disease and support the myeloma cell growth and survival. The better understanding of this biology has revealed several other pathways that enhance osteoclastogenesis, including the PI3K/AKT/mTOR pathway, the extracellular signal-regulated kinase 1/2 pathway, the nuclear export protein CRM1/XPO1 signaling, the MAPK pathways, the parathyroid hormone-related protein, chemokines and their receptors such as the C-C chemokine receptor type 1 and 2 (CCR1 and -2), the C-C motif ligand 3 (CCL-3; previously known as macrophage inflammatory protein 1a) pathways, and others [23, 195–202]. This knowledge has led to the development of novel drugs that may be used in the near future for the management of lytic bone disease in myeloma patients. AKT pathway is upregulated in marrow monocytes from MM patients, leading to a sustained high expression of RANK in osteoclast precursors. AKT inhibition blocks this upregulation of RANK expression and the subsequent osteoclast formation. In the clinical setting, the novel AKT inhibitor LY294002 blocked the formation of myeloma masses in the bone marrow cavity and dramatically reduced osteoclast formation and osteolytic lesions in SCID mice, suggesting a potential role in the management of MM patients with bone disease in the future [196]. AZD6244 is a mitogen-activated or extracellular signal-regulated protein kinase (MEK) inhibitor. It has been reported in preclinical models that AZD6244 blocked osteoclast formation in a dose-dependent manner and inhibited bone resorption targeting a later stage of osteoclast differentiation [197]. Novel, oral, irreversible selective nuclear export inhibitors (SINEs) that target CRM1 have shown strong antimyeloma activity, and they inhibit the MM-induced osteolysis. SINEs have direct anti-osteoclastic function through the blockade of RANKL-induced NF-kB and NFATc1, with almost no impact on osteoblasts, supporting their clinical development for myeloma-related bone disease [198]. MLN3897 is a novel antagonist of the chemokine receptor CCR1 that demonstrated reduction of osteoclast formation and function by inhibiting the AKT signaling and the CCL-3 pathway in preclinical models [203].

8.11 Wnt Pathway Regulators: Helping the Osteoblast

DKK-1 Antagonists. DKK-1 plays an important role in the dysfunction of osteo-blasts observed in MM. The production of this soluble Wnt inhibitor by MM cells inhibits osteoblast activity, and its serum level reflects the extension of focal bone lesions in MM [68, 149]. Serum DKK-1 is increased not only in symptomatic MM patients at diagnosis and but also in relapsed MM, correlating with advanced disease features and the presence of lytic lesions, while serum DKK-1 levels of asymptomatic patients at diagnosis and plateau do not differ from control values [26, 204].

BHQ880, an IgG antibody, the first-in-class, fully human anti-Dkk-1 neutralizing antibody, seems to promote bone formation, and thus it has been shown to inhibit tumor-induced osteolytic disease in preclinical studies [190]. Inhibiting Dkk-1 with BHQ880 in the 5T2MM murine model of myeloma reduced the development of osteolytic bone lesions and in vivo growth of MM cells [205]. A phase I/II study of BHQ880 in combination with zoledronic acid in relapsed or refractory myeloma patients is ongoing as well as phase II studies in patients with high-risk smoldering MM or untreated MM and renal insufficiency. Results are highly anticipated.

Sclerostin Antagonists. Sclerostin is another Wnt inhibitor, specifically expressed by osteocytes, which inhibits osteoblast-driven bone formation and induces mature osteoblast apoptosis [206]. Sclerostin deficiency leads to the development of rare bone sclerosing disorders, including sclerosteosis and van Buchem disease. On the other hand, elevated sclerostin is implicated in the mechanisms of bone loss in metabolic bone diseases, such as postmenopausal osteoporosis and thalassemia-associated osteoporosis [207, 208]. Elevated circulating sclerostin levels correlate with advanced disease features and abnormal bone remodeling in symptomatic myeloma [27]. In particular, MM patients who presented with fractures at diagnosis had very high levels of circulating sclerostin compared with all others ($p < 0.01$), while sclerostin serum levels correlated negatively with bALP ($r = -0.541$; $p < 0.0001$) and positively with CTX ($r = 0.524$; $p < 0.0001$) [27]. Romosozumab (AMG 785; CDP7851), an investigational humanized monoclonal antibody that inhibits the activity of sclerostin, has been used in phase II clinical studies in postmenopausal women with low bone mineral density (BMD), demonstrating significant increases in lumbar spine BMD after 12 months [209]. Studies in MM are planned to start soon.

8.12 Antimyeloma Agents

8.12.1 Bortezomib

Bortezomib is the first proteasome inhibitor with established activity against myeloma, with subsequent effects on osteoclasts that leads to reduced bone resorption [210, 211]. For patients with relapsed/refractory MM, bortezomib reduces circulating RANKL, osteoclast function, and bone resorption, as assessed by TRACP-5b and CTX serum levels, respectively [212]. Furthermore, bortezomib increases osteoblast activity and bone formation both in vitro and for patients with relapsed/refractory MM [213, 214]. More specifically, bortezomib increased bone formation markers such as bALP; this increase was observed both among responders and nonresponders to bortezomib suggesting a direct effect of bortezomib on osteoblastic activity [215]. Another proteasome inhibitor, carfilzomib, has been reported to increase bALP in patients with relapsed/refractory MM that responded to therapy [216]. Bortezomib in combination with zoledronic acid increased BMD in a subset of MM patients at first relapse even in the presence of dexamethasone [217]. However, when bortezomib was given in combination with other antimyeloma drugs, such as melphalan and thalidomide (VMDT regimen), no increase in bALP and osteocalcin was observed suggesting that in such combinations bortezomib seems to lose its beneficial effect on osteoblasts [218]. Even in post-autologous stem cell transplantation patients with low myeloma burden, bortezomib in combination with thalidomide and dexamethasone as consolidation therapy failed to produce a significant bone anabolic effect [219]. Nevertheless, in this specific cohort of patients who did not receive BPs during consolidation, bone resorption was reduced, and there were no SREs in responding patients. In a subanalysis of a phase III study in newly diagnosed patients (VISTA trial), bortezomib in combination with melphalan and prednisone (VMP) reduced substantially DKK-1 in responding patients, while the MP regimen increased DKK-1 even in responders [220]. In the same study, there was evident bone formation effect in conventional radiography in subset of VMP patients but not in MP patients [220].

These findings suggest that proteasome inhibition and especially bortezomib, in addition to its antineoplastic effects on tumor cells, may directly stimulate osteoblast differentiation and function and lead to increased bone formation and increased BMD, at least in responders. However, it is unclear if bortezomib alone is sufficient to reverse bone disease in MM patients and heal lytic lesions as evidence of the effect of bortezomib on clinical end points specific to the bone, such as SREs is limited, possibly as a result of relatively short follow-up periods. Prospective trials that specifically investigate end points related to bone formation are needed.

8.13 Immunomodulatory Agents

Immunomodulatory agents (IMiDs), such as thalidomide, lenalidomide, and pomalidomide, are highly active agents in the treatment of both newly diagnosed and relapsed/refractory MM. These agents also alter interactions between bone marrow microenvironment and malignant plasma cells and modify abnormal bone metabolism in MM [23].

Thalidomide. Thalidomide almost completely blocks RANKL-induced osteoclast formation in vitro. In relapsed/refractory MM patients, intermediate dose of thalidomide (200 mg/day) in combination with dexamethasone produced a significant reduction of serum markers of bone resorption [C-telopeptide of collagen type I (CTX) and tartrate-resistant acid phosphatase isoform-5b (TRACP-5b)] and also of sRANKL/OPG ratio [221].

Lenalidomide. Lenalidomide also inhibited osteoclast formation, by targeting PU.1, a critical transcription factor for the development of osteoclasts, and down-regulating cathepsin K. The downregulation of PU.1 in hematopoietic progenitor cells resulted in a complete shift of lineage development toward granulocytes. Lenalidomide also reduced the serum levels of sRANKL/OPG ratio in MM patients [222].

Pomalidomide. Pomalidomide, like thalidomide, blocks RANKL-induced osteoclastogenesis in vitro, even at concentrations of one µM, which is similar or even lower than that achieved in vivo after the therapeutic administration of this agent. Pomalidomide downregulates transcription factor PU.1, affecting the lineage commitment of osteoclast precursors toward granulocytes instead of mature osteoclasts [223].

8.14   Other Novel Agents

Panobinostat is a histone deacetylase inhibitor, which has shown significant pre-clinical antimyeloma activity and is currently in phase III trials for relapsed MM. Recently, a potent synergistic antiproliferative effect of panobinostat with zoledronic acid was described in three myeloma cell lines and may result in clinical trials in myeloma patients [224].

Bruton's tyrosine kinase (BTK) has been reported to play an important role in myeloma cell homing to bone and the subsequent myeloma-induced bone disease [225]. Several BTK inhibitors have been developed including ibrutinib, which was recently approved for the treatment of mantle cell lymphoma. This new category of drugs has entered into clinical trials in myeloma patients and may be used in the future in patients with bone disease.

Other novel antimyeloma agents have also shown effects on bone disease in pre-clinical models. Antibodies against B cell activating factor (anti-BAFF) have produced direct antimyeloma effects and reductions in tartrate-resistant acid phosphatase-positive osteoclasts and in lytic lesions in anti-BAFF-treated animals [226]. Similarly, SCIO-469, a selective p38a MAPK inhibitor, inhibited MM growth and prevented bone disease in the 5T2MM and 5T33MM animal models [227].

8.15   Kyphoplasty and Vertebroplasty

Several studies have demonstrated that balloon kyphoplasty (BKP) or vertebro-plasty is well-tolerated and effective procedures that provide pain relief and improve functional outcomes in patients with painful neoplastic spinal fractures. A single randomized study of 134 patients with bone metastases due to solid tumors and MM demonstrated that treatment of VCFs with BKP was associated with clinically meaningful improvements in physical functioning, back pain, QoL, and ability to perform daily activities relative to nonsurgical management. These benefits persisted throughout the 12-month study [228]. A meta-analysis of 7 nonrandomized studies of patients with MM or osteolytic metastasis revealed that BKP was associated with reduced pain and improved functional outcomes, benefits that were maintained up to 2 years post-procedure ($N = 306$). BKP also improved early vertebral height loss and spinal deformity, but these effects were not long-term [229]. Similarly, a retrospective review of 67 patients with MM-related vertebral compression fractures (VCFs) demonstrated that vertebroplasty provided clinically meaningful improvements in physical functioning, pain, and mobility throughout 12 months of follow-up [230]. Several small nonrandomized studies of BKP or BKP and vertebroplasty generated comparable results [231–233]. However, the role of vertebroplasty for myeloma patients remains debatable in the absence of prospective data [232, 234], as two randomized trials failed to show any benefit of vertebroplasty in patients with osteoporotic fractures vs. conservative therapy [235, 236]. Furthermore, a meta-analysis of 59 studies (56 case series) showed that BKP appears to be more effective than vertebroplasty in relieving pain secondary to cancer-related VCFs and is associated with lower rates of cement leakage [237].

8.16 Radiation Therapy

Several studies, the majority of which were retrospective and included relatively small patient cohorts, demonstrated that radiotherapy provided pain relief, decreased analgesic use, promoted recalcification, reduced neurologic symptoms, and improved motor function and QoL in patients with MM [238–240]. In addition, the total administered dose should be limited and the field of therapy restricted, especially when the aim of treatment is pain relief rather than treatment or prevention of pathologic fractures. A single 8- to 10-Gy fraction is generally recommended. Indeed, single fractions are increasingly preferred to fractionated treatment. No difference in rapidity of onset or duration of pain relief was observed between a single 8-Gy fraction and a fractionated 2-week course of 30 Gy in a randomized study of 288 patients with widespread bony metastases, including 23 patients with MM [241].

MM accounts for 11% of the most prevalent cancer diagnoses causing spinal cord compression (SCC) [242]. In the largest retrospective series to date, radiotherapy alone improved motor function in 75% of patients with MM and SCC. One-year local control was 100%, and 1-year survival was 94% [243].

8.17 Surgery

Surgery is usually directed toward preventing or repair of axial fractures, unstable spinal fractures, and SCC in myeloma patients. Decompression laminectomy is rarely required in MM patients, but radioresistant MM or retropulsed bone fragments may require surgical intervention [244]. In a relatively large study, 75 MM patients were treated surgically (83 interventions) for skeletal complications of the disease. Most of the lesions were in the axial skeleton or the proximal extremities apart from one distal lesion of the fibula, and most surgery was performed in the spine (35 patients). Surgical treatment in these patients was mostly limited to a palliative approach and was well tolerated [245].

References

1. Kumar SK, Rajkumar SV, Dispenzieri A, et al. Improved survival in multiple myeloma and the impact of novel therapies. Blood. 2008;111:2516–20.
2. Kastritis E, Zervas K, Symeonidis A, et al. Improved survival of patients with multiple myeloma after the introduction of novel agents and the applicability of the International Staging System (ISS): an analysis of the Greek Myeloma Study Group (GMSG). Leukemia. 2009;23:1152–7.
3. Jemal A, Siegel R, Xu J, et al. Cancer statistics. CA Cancer J Clin. 2010;60:277–300.
4. Parker SL, Davis KJ, Wingo PA, et al. Cancer statistics by race and ethnicity. CA Cancer J Clin. 1998;48:31–48.
5. Kyle RA, Gertz MA, Witzig TE, et al. Review of 1027 patients with newly diagnosed multiple myeloma. Mayo Clin Proc. 2003;78:21–33.
6. Terpos E, Dimopoulos MA. Myeloma bone disease: pathophysiology and management. Ann Oncol. 2005;16:1223–31.
7. Raje N, Roodman GD. Advances in the biology and treatment of bone disease in multiple myeloma. Clin Cancer Res. 2011;17:1278–86.
8. Coleman RE. Skeletal complications of malignancy. Cancer. 2007;80:1588–94.
9. Roodman GD. Novel targets for myeloma bone disease. Expert Opin Ther Targets. 2008;12:1377–87.
10. Croucher PI, Apperley JF. Bone disease in multiple myeloma. Br J Haematol. 1998;103:902–10.
11. Cocks K, Cohen D, Wisloff F, et al. An international field study of the reliability and validity of a disease-specific questionnaire module (the QLQ-MY20) in assessing the quality of life of patients with multiple myeloma. Eur J Cancer. 2007;43:1670–8.
12. Bruce NJ, McCloskey EV, Kanis JA, et al. Economic impact of using clodronate in the management of patients with multiple myeloma. Br J Haematol. 1999;104:358–64.
13. McCloskey EV, MacLennan IC, Drayson MT, et al. A randomized trial of the effect of clodronate on skeletal morbidity in multiple myeloma. MRC Working Party on Leukaemia in Adults. Br J Haematol. 1998;100:317–25.
14. Rajkumar SV, Dimopoulos MA, Palumbo A, et al. International Myeloma Working Group updated criteria for the diagnosis of multiple myeloma. Lancet Oncol. 2014;15:e538–48.
15. Silbermann R, Roodman GD. Current controversies in the management of myeloma bone disease. J Cell Physiol. 2016; doi:10.1002/jcp.25351. [Epub ahead of print].
16. Bataille R, Chappard D, Marcelli C, et al. Recruitment of new osteoblasts and osteoclasts is the earliest critical event in the pathogenesis of human multiple myeloma. J Clin Invest. 1991;88(1):62–6.
17. Abe M, Hiura K, Wilde J, et al. Osteoclasts enhance myeloma cell growth and survival via cell-cell contact: a vicious cycle between bone destruction and myeloma expansion. Blood. 2004;104(8):2484–91.
18. Tanaka Y, Abe M, Hiasa M, et al. Myeloma cell-osteoclast interaction enhances angiogenesis together with bone resorption: a role for vascular endothelial cell growth factor and osteopontin. Clin Cancer Res. 2007;13(3):816–23.
19. Pearse RN, Sordillo EM, Yaccoby S, et al. Multiple myeloma disrupts the TRANCE/osteoprotegerin cytokine axis to trigger bone destruction and promote tumor progression. Proc Natl Acad Sci U S A. 2001;98:11581–6.
20. Terpos E, Szydlo R, Apperley JF, et al. Soluble receptor activator of nuclear factor kappaB ligand-osteoprotegerin ratio predicts survival in multiple myeloma: proposal for a novel prognostic index. Blood. 2003;102:1064–9.

21. Sugatani T, Alvarez UM, Hruska KA. Activin A stimulates IkappaB-alpha/NFkappaB and RANK expression for osteoclast differentiation, but not AKT survival pathway in osteoclast precursors. J Cell Biochem. 2003;90:59–67.

22. Terpos E, Kastritis E, Christoulas D, et al. Circulating activin-A is elevated in patients with advanced multiple myeloma and correlates with extensive bone involvement and inferior survival; no alterations post-lenalidomide and dexamethasone therapy. Ann Oncol. 2012;23:2681–6.

23. Christoulas D, Terpos E, Dimopoulos MA. Pathogenesis and management of myeloma bone disease. Expert Rev Hematol. 2009;2:385–98.

24. Tian E, Zhan F, Walker R, et al. The role of the Wnt-signaling antagonist DKK1 in the development of osteolytic lesions in multiple myeloma. N Engl J Med. 2003;349:2483–94.

25. Colucci S, Brunetti G, Oranger A, et al. Myeloma cells suppress osteoblasts through sclerostin secretion. Blood Cancer J. 2011;1:e27.

26. Politou MC, Heath DJ, Rahemtulla A, et al. Serum concentrations of Dickkopf-1 protein are increased in patients with multiple myeloma and reduced after autologous stem cell transplantation. Int J Cancer. 2006;119:1728–31.

27. Terpos E, Christoulas D, Katodritou E, et al. Elevated circulating sclerostin correlates with advanced disease features and abnormal bone remodeling in symptomatic myeloma: reduction post-bortezomib monotherapy. Int J Cancer. 2012;131:1466–71.

28. Oshima T, Abe M, Asano J, et al. Myeloma cells suppress bone formation by secreting a soluble Wnt inhibitor, sFRP-2. Blood. 2005;106:3160–5.

29. Dimopoulos M, Terpos E, Comenzo RL, et al. International myeloma working group consensus statement and guidelines regarding the current role of imaging techniques in the diagnosis and monitoring of multiple Myeloma. Leukemia. 2009;23:1545–56.

30. Terpos E, Moulopoulos LA, Dimopoulos MA. Advances in imaging and the management of myeloma bone disease. J Clin Oncol. 2011;29:1907–15.

31. Pianko MJ, Terpos E, Roodman GD, et al. Whole-body low-dose computed tomography and advanced imaging techniques for multiple myeloma bone disease. Clin Cancer Res. 2014;20:5888–97.

32. Ippolito D, Besostri V, Bonaffini PA, et al. Diagnostic value of whole-body low-dose computed tomography (WBLDCT) in bone lesions detection in patients with multiple myeloma. Eur J Radiol. 2013;82:2322–7.

33. Horger M, Claussen CD, Bross-Bach U, et al. Whole-body low-dose multidetector row-CT in the diagnosis of multiple myeloma: an alternative to conventional radiography. Eur J Radiol. 2005;54:289–97.

34. Kropil P, Fenk R, Fritz LB, et al. Comparison of whole- body 64-slice multidetector computed tomography and conventional radiography in staging of multiple myeloma. Eur Radiol. 2008;18:51–8.

35. Gleeson TG, Moriarty J, Shortt CP, et al. Accuracy of whole-body low-dose multidetector CT (WBLDCT) versus skeletal survey in the detection of myelomatous lesions, and correlation of disease distribution with whole-body MRI (WBMRI). Skelet Radiol. 2009;38:225–36.

36. Princewill K, Kyere S, Awan O, et al. Multiple myeloma lesion detection with whole body CT versus radiographic skeletal survey. Cancer Investig. 2013;31:206–11.

37. Wolf MB, Murray F, Kilk K, et al. Sensitivity of whole-body CT and MRI versus projection radiography in the detection of osteolyses in patients with monoclonal plasma cell disease. Eur J Radiol. 2014;83:1222–30.

38. Cretti F, Perugini G. Patient dose evaluation for the whole-body low-dose multidetector CT (WBLDMDCT) skeleton study in multiple myeloma (MM). Radiol Med. 2016;121(2):93–105.

39. Borggrefe J, Giravent S, Campbell G, et al. Association of osteolytic lesions, bone mineral loss and trabecular sclerosis with prevalent vertebral fractures in patients with multiple myeloma. Eur J Radiol. 2015;84:2269–74.

40. Terpos E, Kleber M, Engelhardt M, et al. European Myeloma Network guidelines for the management of multiple myeloma-related complications. Haematologica. 2015;100:1254–66.

41. Moulopoulos LA, Dimopoulos MA. Magnetic resonance imaging of the bone marrow in hematologic malignancies. Blood. 1997;90:2127–47.

42. Libshitz HI, Malthouse SR, Cunningham D, et al. Multiple myeloma: appearance at MR imaging. Radiology. 1992;182:833–7.
43. Weininger M, Lauterbach B, Knop S, et al. Whole-body MRI of multiple myeloma: comparison of different MRI sequences in assessment of different growth patterns. Eur J Radiol. 2008;69:339–45.
44. Attariwala R, Picker W. Whole body MRI: improved lesion detection and characterization with diffusion weighted techniques. J Magn Reson Imaging. 2013;38:253–68.
45. Muller MF, Edelman RR. Echo planar imaging of the abdomen. Top Magn Reson Imaging. 1995;7:112–9.
46. Wang Y. Description of parallel imaging in MRI using multiple coils. Magn Reson Med. 2000;44:495–9.
47. Nonomura Y, Yasumoto M, Yoshimura R, et al. Relationship between bone marrow cellularity and apparent diffusion coefficient. J Magn Reson Imaging. 2001;13:757–60.
48. Terpos E, Koutoulidis V, Fontara S, et al. Diffusion-weighted imaging improves accuracy in the diagnosis of MRI patterns of marrow involvement in newly diagnosed myeloma: results of a prospective study in 99 patients. Blood. 2015;126:4178 (ASH abstract).
49. Xu X, Ma L, Zhang JS, et al. Feasibility of whole body diffusion weighted imaging in detecting bone metastasis on 3.0T MR scanner. Chin Med Sci J. 2008;23:151–7.
50. Messiou C, Giles S, Collins DJ, et al. Assessing response of myeloma bone disease with diffusion-weighted MRI. Br J Radiol. 2012;85:e1198–203.
51. Messiou C, Collins DJ, Morgan VA, et al. Optimizing diffusion weighted MRI for imaging metastatic and myeloma bone disease and assessing reproducibility. Eur Radiol. 2011;21:1713–8.
52. Hillengass J, Bäuerle T, Bartl R, et al. Diffusion-weighted imaging for non-invasive and quantitative monitoring of bone marrow infiltration in patients with monoclonal plasma cell disease: a comparative study with histology. Br J Haematol. 2011;153:721–8.
53. Lemke A, Stieltjes B, Schad LR, et al. Toward an optimal distribution of b values for intra-voxel incoherent motion imaging. Magn Reson Imaging. 2011;29:766–76.
54. Giles SL, deSouza NM, Collins DJ, et al. Assessing myeloma bone disease with whole-body diffusion-weighted imaging: comparison with x-ray skeletal survey by region and relationship with laboratory estimates of disease burden. Clin Radiol. 2015;70:614–21.
55. Sachpekidis C, Mosebach J, Freitag MT, et al. Application of (18)F-FDG PET and diffusion weighted imaging (DWI) in multiple myeloma: comparison of functional imaging modalities. Am J Nucl Med Mol Imaging. 2015;5:479–92.
56. Pawlyn C, Fowkes L, Otero S, et al. Whole-body diffusion-weighted MRI: a new gold standard for assessing disease burden in patients with multiple myeloma? Leukemia leu. 2015;2015:338. doi:10.1038/leu.2015.338.
57. Horger M, Weisel K, Horger W, et al. Whole-body diffusion-weighted MRI with apparent diffusion coefficient mapping for early response monitoring in multiple myeloma: preliminary results. AJR Am J Roentgenol. 2011;196:W790–5.
58. Hillengass J, Wasser K, Delorme S, et al. Lumbar bone marrow microcirculation measurements from dynamic contrast-enhanced magnetic resonance imaging is a predictor of event-free survival in progressive multiple myeloma. Clin Cancer Res. 2007;13:475–81.
59. Hillengass J, Landgren O. Challenges and opportunities of novel imaging techniques in monoclonal plasma cell disorders: imaging "early myeloma". Leuk Lymphoma. 2013;54:1355–63.
60. Huang SY, Chen BB, HY L, et al. Correlation among DCE-MRI measurements of bone marrow angiogenesis, microvessel density, and extramedullary disease in patients with multiple myeloma. Am J Hematol. 2012;87:837–9.
61. Zechmann CM, Traine L, Meissner T, et al. Parametric histogram analysis of dynamic contrast-enhanced MRI in multiple myeloma: a technique to evaluate angiogenic response to therapy? Acad Radiol. 2012;19:100–8.
62. Zwick S, Brix G, Tofts PS, et al. Simulation-based comparison of two approaches frequently used for dynamic contrast-enhanced MRI. Eur Radiol. 2010;20:432–42.

63. Fraioli F, Punwani S. Clinical and research applications of simultaneous positron emission tomography and MRI. Br J Radiol. 2014;87:20130464.
64. Sachpekidis C, Hillengass J, Goldschmidt H, et al. Comparison of (18)F-FDG PET/CT and PET/MRI in patients with multiple myeloma. Am J Nucl Med Mol Imaging. 2015;5:469–78.
65. Baur-Melnyk A, Buhmann S, Durr HR, et al. Role of MRI for the diagnosis and prognosis of multiple myeloma. Eur J Radiol. 2005;55:56–63.
66. Moulopoulos LA, Varma DG, Dimopoulos MA, et al. Multiple myeloma: spinal MR imaging in patients with untreated newly diagnosed disease. Radiology. 1992;185:833–40.
67. Moulopoulos LA, Gika D, Anagnostopoulos A, et al. Prognostic significance of magnetic resonance imaging of bone marrow in previously untreated patients with multiple myeloma. Ann Oncol. 2005;16:1824–8.
68. Durie BGM. The role of anatomic and functional staging in myeloma: description of Durie/ Salmon plus staging system. Eur J Cancer. 2006;42:1539–43.
69. Walker R, Barlogie B, Haessler J, et al. Magnetic resonance imaging in multiple myeloma: diagnostic and clinical implications. J Clin Oncol. 2007;25:1121–8.
70. Ludwig H, Frühwald F, Tscholakoff D, et al. Magnetic resonance imaging of the spine in multiple myeloma. Lancet. 1987;2:364–6.
71. Ghanem N, Lohrmann C, Engelhardt M, et al. Whole-body MRI in the detection of bone marrow infiltration in patients with plasma cell neoplasms in comparison to the radiological skeletal survey. Eur Radiol. 2006;16:1005–14.
72. Lecouvet FE, Malghem J, Michaux L, et al. Skeletal survey in advanced multiple myeloma: radiographic versus MR imaging survey. Br J Haematol. 1999;106:35–9.
73. Tertti R, Alanen A, Remes K. The value of magnetic resonance imaging in screening myeloma lesions of the lumbar spine. Br J Haematol. 1995;91:658–60.
74. Narquin S, Ingrand P, Azais I, et al. Comparison of whole-body diffusion MRI and conventional radiological assessment in the staging of myeloma. Diagn Interv Imaging. 2013;94:629–36.
75. Regelink JC, Minnema MC, Terpos E, et al. Comparison of modern and conventional imaging techniques in establishing multiple myeloma-related bone disease: a systematic review. Br J Haematol. 2013;162:50–61.
76. Baur-Melnyk A, Buhmann S, Becker C, et al. Whole-body MRI versus whole-body MDCT for staging of multiple myeloma. AJR Am J Roentgenol. 2008;190:1097–104.
77. Zamagni E, Nanni C, Patriarca F, et al. A prospective comparison of 18F-fluorodeoxyglucose positron emission tomography-computed tomography, magnetic resonance imaging and whole-body planar radiographs in the assessment of bone disease in newly diagnosed multiple myeloma. Haematologica. 2007;92:50–5.
78. Waheed S, Mitchell A, Usmani S, et al. Standard and novel imaging methods for multiple myeloma: correlates with prognostic laboratory variables including gene expression profiling data. Haematologica. 2013;98:71–8.
79. Khalafallah AA, Snarski A, Heng R, et al. Assessment of whole body MRI and sestamibi technetium-99m bone marrow scan in prediction of multiple myeloma disease progression and outcome: a prospective comparative study. BMJ Open. 2013;3:e002025.
80. Bauerle T, Hillengass J, Fechtner K, et al. Multiple myeloma and monoclonal gammopathy of undetermined significance: importance of whole-body versus spinal MR imaging. Radiology. 2009;252:477–85.
81. Baur A, Stabler A, Bruning R, et al. Diffusion-weighted MR imaging of bone marrow: differentiation of benign versus pathologic compression fractures. Radiology. 1998;207:349–56.
82. Moulopoulos LA, Dimopoulos MA, Weber D, et al. Magnetic resonance imaging in the staging of solitary plasmacytoma of bone. J Clin Oncol. 1993;11:1311–5.
83. Dimopoulos MA, Moulopoulos LA, Maniatis A, et al. Solitary plasmacytoma of bone and asymptomatic multiple myeloma. Blood. 2000;96:2037–44.
84. Varettoni M, Corso A, Pica G, et al. Incidence, presenting features and outcome of extramedullary disease in multiple myeloma: a longitudinal study on 1003 consecutive patients. Ann Oncol. 2010;21:325–30.

85. Lafforgue P, Dahan E, Chagnaud C, et al. Early-stage avascular necrosis of the femoral head: MR imaging for prognosis in 31 cases with at least 2 years of follow-up. Radiology. 1993;187:199–204.
86. Syed IS, Glockner JF, Feng D, et al. Role of cardiac magnetic resonance imaging in the detection of cardiac amyloidosis. JACC Cardiovasc Imaging. 2010;3:155–64.
87. Carlson K, Aström G, Nyman R, et al. MR imaging of multiple myeloma in tumour mass measurement at diagnosis and during treatment. Acta Radiol. 1995;36:9–14.
88. Dimopoulos MA, Hillengass J, Usmani S, et al. Role of magnetic resonance imaging in the management of patients with multiple myeloma: a consensus statement. J Clin Oncol. 2015;33(6):657–64. doi:10.1200/JCO.2014.57.9961.
89. Usmani SZ, Mitchell A, Waheed S, et al. Prognostic implications of serial 18-fluoro-deoxyglucose emission tomography in multiple myeloma treated with total therapy. Blood. 2013;121:1819–23.
90. Lecouvet FE, Vande Berg BC, Michaux L, et al. Stage III multiple myeloma: clinical and prognostic value of spinal bone marrow MR imaging. Radiology. 1998;209:653–60.
91. Moulopoulos LA, Dimopoulos MA, Kastritis E, et al. Diffuse pattern of bone marrow involvement on magnetic resonance imaging is associated with high risk cytogenetics and poor outcome in newly diagnosed, symptomatic patients with multiple myeloma: a single center experience on 228 patients. Am J Hematol. 2012;87:861–4.
92. Moulopoulos LA, Dimopoulos MA, Christoulas D, et al. Diffuse MRI marrow pattern correlates with increased angiogenesis, advanced disease features and poor prognosis in newly diagnosed myeloma treated with novel agents. Leukemia. 2010;24:1206–12.
93. Song MK, Chung JS, Lee JJ, et al. Magnetic resonance imaging pattern of bone marrow involvement as a new predictive parameter of disease progression in newly diagnosed patients with multiple myeloma eligible for autologous stem cell transplantation. Br J Haematol. 2014;165(6):777–85. doi:10.1111/bjh.12820.
94. Moulopoulos LA, Dimopoulos MA, Alexanian R, et al. Multiple myeloma: MR patterns of response to treatment. Radiology. 1994;193:441–6.
95. Hillengass J, Ayyaz S, Kilk K, et al. Changes in magnetic resonance imaging before and after autologous stem cell transplantation correlate with response and survival in multiple myeloma. Haematologica. 2012;97:1757–60.
96. Bannas P, Hentschel HB, Bley TA, et al. Diagnostic performance of whole-body MRI for the detection of persistent or relapsing disease in multiple myeloma after stem cell transplantation. Eur Radiol. 2012;22:2007–12.
97. Derlin T, Peldschus K, Münster S, et al. Comparative diagnostic performance of ^{18}F-FDG PET/CT versus whole-body MRI for determination of remission status in multiple myeloma after stem cell transplantation. Eur Radiol. 2013;23:570–8.
98. Spinnato P, Bazzocchi A, Brioli A, et al. Contrast enhanced MRI and ^{18}F-FDG PET-CT in the assessment of multiple myeloma: a comparison of results in different phases of the disease. Eur J Radiol. 2012;81:4013–8.
99. Bartel TB, Haessler J, Brown TL, et al. F18-fluorodeoxyglucose positron emission tomography in the context of other imaging techniques and prognostic factors in multiple myeloma. Blood. 2009;114:2068–76.
100. Giles SL, Messiou C, Collins DJ, et al. Whole-body diffusion-weighted MR imaging for assessment of treatment response in Myeloma. Radiology. 2014;271(3):785–94.
101. Dimopoulos MA, Moulopoulos A, Smith T, et al. Risk of disease progression in asymptomatic multiple myeloma. Am J Med. 1993;94:57–61.
102. Moulopoulos LA, Dimopoulos MA, Smith TL, et al. Prognostic significance of magnetic resonance imaging in patients with asymptomatic multiple myeloma. J Clin Oncol. 1995;13:251–6.
103. Hillengass J, Fechtner K, Weber MA, et al. Prognostic significance of focal lesions in whole-body magnetic resonance imaging in patients with asymptomatic multiple myeloma. J Clin Oncol. 2010;28:1606–10.

104. Kastritis E, Terpos E, Moulopoulos L, et al. Extensive bone marrow infiltration and abnormal free light chain ratio identifies patients with asymptomatic myeloma at high risk for progression to symptomatic disease. Leukemia. 2013;27:947–53.

105. Merz M, Hielscher T, Wagner B, et al. Predictive value of longitudinal whole-body magnetic resonance imaging in patients with smoldering multiple myeloma. Leukemia. 2014;28(9):1902–8.

106. Pepe J, Petrucci MT, Nofroni I, et al. Lumbar bone mineral density as the major factor determining increased prevalence of vertebral fractures in monoclonal gammopathy of undetermined significance. Br J Haematol. 2006;134:485–90.

107. Van de Donk NW, Palumbo A, Johnsen HE, et al. The clinical relevance and management of monoclonal gammopathy of undetermined significance and related disorders: recommendations from the European Myeloma Network. Haematologica. 2014;99(6):984–96.

108. Vande Berg BC, Michaux L, Lecouvet FE, et al. Nonmyelomatous monoclonal gammopathy: correlation of bone marrow MR images with laboratory findings and spontaneous clinical outcome. Radiology. 1997;202:247–51.

109. Dhodapkar MV, Sexton R, Waheed S, et al. Clinical, genomic, and imaging predictors of myeloma progression from asymptomatic monoclonal gammopathies (SWOG S0120). Blood. 2014;123:78–85.

110. Hillengass J, Weber MA, Kilk K, et al. Prognostic significance of whole-body MRI in patients with monoclonal gammopathy of undetermined significance. Leukemia. 2014;28:174–8.

111. Liebross RH, Ha CS, Cox JD, et al. Solitary bone plasmacytoma: outcome and prognostic factors following radiotherapy. Int J Radiat Oncol Biol Phys. 1998;41:1063–7.

112. Bredella MA, Steinbach L, Caputo G, et al. Value of FDG PET in the assessment of patients with multiple myeloma. AJR Am J Roentgenol. 2005;184:1199–204.

113. Lütje S, de Rooy JW, Croockewit S, et al. Role of radiography, MRI and FDG-PET/CT in diagnosing, staging and therapeutical evaluation of patients with multiple myeloma. Ann Hematol. 2009;88:1161–8.

114. Breyer RJ 3rd, Mulligan ME, Smith SE, et al. Comparison of imaging with FDG PET/CT with other imaging modalities in myeloma. Skeletal Radiol. 2006;35:632–40.

115. Zamagni E, Nanni C, Gay F, et al. 18F-FDG PET/CT focal, but not osteolytic, lesions predict the progression of smoldering myeloma to active disease. Leukemia. 2015;30(2):417–22. doi:10.1038/leu.2015.291.

116. Siontis B, Kumar S, Dispenzieri A, et al. Positron emission tomography-computed tomography in the diagnostic evaluation of smoldering multiple myeloma: identification of patients needing therapy. Blood Cancer J. 2015;5:e364.

117. Sachpekidis C, Mai EK, Goldschmidt H, et al. (18)F-FDG dynamic PET/CT in patients with multiple myeloma: patterns of tracer uptake and correlation with bone marrow plasma cell infiltration rate. Clin Nucl Med. 2015;40:e300–7.

118. Tirumani SH, Sakellis C, Jacene H, et al. Role of FDG-PET/CT in extramedullary multiple myeloma: correlation of FDG-PET/CT findings with clinical outcome. Clin Nucl Med. 2016;41:e7–e13.

119. Zamagni E, Nanni C, Mancuso K, et al. PET/CT improves the definition of complete response and allows to detect otherwise unidentifiable skeletal progression in multiple myeloma. Clin Cancer Res. 2015;21:4384–90.

120. Paiva B, van Dongen JJ, Orfao A, et al. New criteria for response assessment: role of minimal residual disease in multiple myeloma. Blood. 2015;125:3059–68.

121. Zamagni E, Patriarca F, Nanni C, et al. Prognostic relevance of 18-F FDG PET/CT in newly diagnosed multiple myeloma patients treated with up-front autologous transplantation. Blood. 2011;118:5989–95.

122. Patriarca F, Carobolante F, Zamagni E, et al. The role of positron emission tomography with 18F-fluorodeoxyglucose integrated with computed tomography in the evaluation of patients with multiple myeloma undergoing allogeneic stem cell transplantation. Biol Blood Marrow Transplant. 2015;21:1068–73.

123. Fonti R, Pace L, Cerchione C, et al. 18F-FDG PET/CT, 99mTc-MIBI, and MRI in the prediction of outcome of patients with multiple myeloma: a comparative study. Clin Nucl Med. 2015;40:303–8.
124. Lapa C, Lückerath K, Malzahn U, et al. 18 FDG-PET/CT for prognostic stratification of patients with multiple myeloma relapse after stem cell transplantation. Oncotarget. 2014;5(17):7381–91.
125. Cascini GL, Falcone C, Console D, et al. Whole-body MRI and PET/CT in multiple myeloma patients during staging and after treatment: personal experience in a longitudinal study. Radiol Med. 2013;118(6):930–48.
126. Moreau P, Attal M, Karlin L, et al. Prospective evaluation of MRI and PET-CT at diagnosis and before maintenance therapy in symptomatic patients with Multiple Myeloma included in the IFM/DFCI 2009 trial. Blood. 2015;126:395 (ASH abstract).
127. Nanni C, Zamagni E, Versari A, et al. Image interpretation criteria for FDG PET/CT in multiple myeloma: a new proposal from an Italian expert panel. IMPeTUs (Italian Myeloma criteria for PET USe). Eur J Nucl Med Mol Imaging. 2016;43:414–21.
128. Fouquet G, Guidez S, Herbaux C, et al. Impact of initial FDG-PET/CT and serum-free light chain on transformation of conventionally defined solitary plasmacytoma to multiple myeloma. Clin Cancer Res. 2014;20:3254–60.
129. Alongi P, Zanoni L, Incerti E, et al. 18F-FDG PET/CT for early post-radiotherapy assessment in solitary bone plasmacytomas. Clin Nucl Med. 2015;40:e399–404.
130. Lonial S, Kaufman JL. Non-secretory myeloma: a clinician's guide. Oncology (Williston Park). 2013;27:924–8.
131. Rogers MJ, Gordon S, Benford HL, et al. Cellular and molecular mechanisms of action of bisphosphonates. Cancer. 2000;88:2961.
132. Terpos E, Sezer O, Croucher PI, et al. The use of bisphosphonates in multiple myeloma recommendations of an expert panel on behalf of the European Myeloma Network. Ann Oncol. 2009;20:1303.
133. Boonekamp PM, van der Wee-Pals LJ, van Wijk-van Lennep MM, et al. Two modes of action of bisphosphonates on osteoclastic resorption of mineralized matrix. Bone Miner. 1986;1:27.
134. Rowe DJ, Etre LA, Lovdahl MJ, et al. Relationship between bisphosphonate concentration and osteoclast activity and viability. In Vitro Cell Dev Biol Anim. 1999;35:383.
135. Terpos E, Berenson J, Raje N, et al. Management of bone disease in multiple myeloma. Expert Rev Hematol. 2014;7(1):113–25.
136. Mundy GR, Yoneda T. Bisphosphonates as anticancer drugs. N Engl J Med. 1998;339:398.
137. Yin JJ, Selander K, Chirgwin JM, et al. TGF-beta signaling blockade inhibits PTHrP secretion by breast cancer cells and bone metastases development. J Clin Invest. 1999;103:197.
138. Diel IJ, Solomayer EF, Costa SD, et al. Reduction in new metastases in breast cancer with adjuvant clodronate treatment. N Engl J Med. 1998;339:357.
139. Aparicio A, Gardner A, Tu Y, et al. In vitro cytoreductive effects on multiple myeloma cells induced by bisphosphonates. Leukemia. 1998;12:220.
140. Shipman CM, Rogers MJ, Apperley JF, et al. Bisphosphonates induce apoptosis in human myeloma cell lines: a novel anti-tumour activity. Br J Haematol. 1997;98:665.
141. Dhodapkar MV, Singh J, Mehta J, et al. Anti-myeloma activity of pamidronate in vivo. Br J Haematol. 1998;103:530.
142. Daragon A, Humez C, Michot C, et al. Treatment of multiple myeloma with etidronate: results of a multicentre double-blind study. Eur J Med. 1993;2(8):449–52.
143. Menssen HD, Sakalova A, Fontana A, et al. Effects of long-term intravenous ibandronate therapy on skeletal-related events, survival, and bone resorption markers in patients with advanced multiple myeloma. J Clin Oncol. 2002;20(9):2353–9.
144. Terpos E, Morgan G, all DMA e. International Myeloma Working Group recommendations for the treatment of multiple myeloma-related bone disease. J Clin Oncol. 2013;31(18):2347–57.
145. Belch AR, Bergsagel DE, Wilson K, et al. Effect of daily etidronate on the osteolysis of multiple myeloma. J Clin Oncol. 1991;9(8):1397–402.

146. Lahtinen R, Laakso M, Palva I, et al. Randomised, placebo-controlled multicentre trial of clodronate in multiple myeloma. Lancet. 1992;340(8832):1049–52.
147. McCloskey EV, Dunn JA, Kanis JA, et al. Long-term follow-up of a prospective, double-blind, placebo-controlled randomized trial of clodronate in multiple myeloma. Br J Haematol. 2001;113(4):1035–43.
148. Berenson JR, Lichtenstein A, Porter L, et al. Long-term pamidronate treatment of advanced multiple myeloma patients reduces skeletal events. Myeloma Aredia Study Group. J Clin Oncol. 1998;16(2):593–602.
149. Brincker H, Westin J, Abildgaard N, et al. Failure of oral pamidronate to reduce skeletal morbidity in multiple myeloma: a double-blind placebo-controlled trial. Danish-Swedish co-operative study group. Br J Haematol. 1998;101(2):280–6.
150. Gimsing P, Carlson K, Turesson I, et al. Effect of pamidronate 30 mg versus 90 mg on physical function in patients with newly diagnosed multiple myeloma (Nordic Myeloma Study Group): a double-blind, randomised controlled trial. Lancet Oncol. 2010;11(10):973–82.
151. Berenson JR, Rosen LS, Howell A, et al. Zoledronic acid reduces skeletal-related events in patients with osteolytic metastases. Cancer. 2001;91(7):1191–200.
152. Rosen LS, Gordon D, Kaminski M, et al. Zoledronic acid versus pamidronate in the treatment of skeletal metastases in patients with breast cancer or osteolytic lesions of multiple myeloma: a phase III, double-blind, comparative trial. Cancer J. 2001;7(5):377–87.
153. Rosen LS, Gordon D, Kaminski M, et al. Long-term efficacy and safety of zoledronic acid compared with pamidronate disodium in the treatment of skeletal complications in patients with advanced multiple myeloma or breast carcinoma: a randomized, double-blind, multi-center, comparative trial. Cancer. 2003;98(8):1735–44.
154. Morgan GJ, Davies FE, Gregory WM, et al. First-line treatment with zoledronic acid as compared with clodronic acid in multiple myeloma (MRC Myeloma IX): a randomised controlled trial. Lancet. 2010;376(9757):1989–99.
155. Morgan GJ, Davies FE, Gregory WM, et al. Effects of induction and maintenance plus long-term bisphosphonates on bone disease in patients with multiple myeloma: MRC Myeloma IX trial. Blood. 2012;119(23):5374–83.
156. Croucher PI, De Hendrik R, Perry MJ, et al. Zoledronic acid treatment of 5T2MM-bearing mice inhibits the development of myeloma bone disease: evidence for decreased osteolysis, tumor burden and angiogenesis, and increased survival. J Bone Miner Res. 2003;18(3):482–92.
157. Mhaskar R, Redzepovic J, Wheatley K, et al. Bisphosphonates in multiple myeloma: a network meta-analysis. Cochrane Database Syst Rev. 2012;5:CD003188.
158. D'Arena G, Gobbi PG, Broglia C, et al. Pamidronate versus observation in asymptomatic myeloma: final results with long-term follow-up of a randomized study. Leuk Lymphoma. 2011;52:771–5.
159. Musto P, Petrucci MT, Bringhen S, et al. A multicenter, randomized clinical trial comparing zoledronic acid versus observation in patients with asymptomatic myeloma. Cancer. 2008;113:1588–95.
160. Bida JP, Kyle RA, Therneau TM, et al. Disease associations with monoclonal gammopathy of undetermined significance: a population-based study of 17,398 patients. Mayo Clin Proc. 2009;84:685–93.
161. Kristinsson SY, Tang M, Pfeiffer RM, et al. Monoclonal gammopathy of undetermined significance and risk of skeletal fractures: a population-based study. Blood. 2010;116:2651–5.
162. Berenson JR, Yellin O, Boccia RV, et al. Zoledronic acid markedly improves bone mineral density for patients with monoclonal gammopathy of undetermined significance and bone loss. Clin Cancer Res. 2008;14:6289–95.
163. Pepe J, Petrucci MT, Mascia ML, et al. The effects of alendronate treatment in osteoporotic patients affected by monoclonal gammopathy of undetermined significance. Calcif Tissue Int. 2008;82:418–26.
164. Fechtner K, Hillengass J, Delorme S, et al. Staging monoclonal plasma cell disease: comparison of the Durie-Salmon and the Durie-Salmon PLUS staging systems. Radiology. 2010;257:195–204.

165. Cramer JA, Gold DT, Silverman SL, et al. A systematic review of persistence and compliance with bisphosphonates for osteoporosis. Osteoporos Int. 2007;18:1023–31.
166. Morgan GJ, Child JA, Gregory WM, et al. Effects of zoledronic acid versus clodronic acid on skeletal morbidity in patients with newly diagnosed multiple myeloma (MRC Myeloma IX): secondary outcomes from a randomised controlled trial. Lancet Oncol. 2011;12:743–52.
167. Roux S, Bergot C, Fermand JP, et al. Evaluation of bone mineral density and fat-lean distribution in patients with multiple myeloma in sustained remission. J Bone Miner Res. 2003;18:231–6.
168. Badros A, Goloubeva O, Terpos E, et al. Prevalence and significance of vitamin D deficiency in multiple myeloma patients. Br J Haematol. 2008;142:492–4.
169. Laroche M, Lemaire O, Attal M. Vitamin D deficiency does not alter biochemical markers of bone metabolism before or after autograft in patients with multiple myeloma. Eur J Haematol. 2010;85:65–7.
170. Ross AC, Manson JE, Abrams SA, et al. The 2011 report on dietary reference intakes for calcium and vitamin D from the Institute of Medicine: what clinicians need to know. J Clin Endocrinol Metab. 2011;96:53–8.
171. Berenson JR, Lichtenstein A, Porter L, et al. Efficacy of pamidronate in reducing skeletal events in patients with advanced multiple myeloma. Myeloma Aredia Study Group. N Engl J Med. 1996;334(8):488–93.
172. Bamias A, Kastritis E, Bamia C, et al. Osteonecrosis of the jaw in cancer after treatment with bisphosphonates: incidence and risk factors. J Clin Oncol. 2005;23(34):8580–7.
173. Dimopoulos MA, Kastritis E, Anagnostopoulos A, et al. Osteonecrosis of the jaw in patients with multiple myeloma treated with bisphosphonates: evidence of increased risk after treatment with zoledronic acid. Haematologica. 2006;91(7):968–71.
174. Zervas K, Verrou E, Teleioudis Z, et al. Incidence, risk factors and management of osteonecrosis of the jaw in patients with multiple myeloma: a single-centre experience in 303 patients. Br J Haematol. 2006;134(6):620–3.
175. Badros A, Terpos E, Katodritou E, et al. Natural history of osteonecrosis of the jaw in patients with multiple myeloma. J Clin Oncol. 2008;26(36):5904–9.
176. Coleman RE, Major P, Lipton A, et al. Predictive value of bone resorption and formation markers in cancer patients with bone metastases receiving the bisphosphonate zoledronic acid. J Clin Oncol. 2005;23(22):4925–35.
177. Dimopoulos MA, Kastritis E, Bamia C, et al. Reduction of osteonecrosis of the jaw (ONJ) after implementation of preventive measures in patients with multiple myeloma treated with zoledronic acid. Ann Oncol. 2009;20(1):117–20.
178. Montefusco V, Gay F, Spina F, et al. Antibiotic prophylaxis before dental procedures may reduce the incidence of osteonecrosis of the jaw in patients with multiple myeloma treated with bisphosphonates. Leuk Lymphoma. 2008;49(11):2156–62.
179. Migliorati CA, Casiglia J, Epstein J, et al. Managing the care of patients with bisphosphonate-associated osteonecrosis: an American Academy of Oral Medicine position paper. J Am Dent Assoc. 2005;136(12):1658–68.
180. Ripamonti CI, Cislaghi E, Mariani L, et al. Efficacy and safety of medical ozone (O(3)) delivered in oil suspension applications for the treatment of osteonecrosis of the jaw in patients with bone metastases treated with bisphosphonates: preliminary results of a phase I-II study. Oral Oncol. 2011;47(3):185–90.
181. Agrillo A, Filiaci F, Ramieri V, et al. Bisphosphonate-related osteonecrosis of the jaw (BRONJ): 5 year experience in the treatment of 131 cases with ozone therapy. Eur Rev Med Pharmacol Sci. 2012;16(12):1741–7.
182. Yaccoby S, Pearse RN, Johnson CL, et al. Myeloma interacts with the bone marrow microenvironment to induce osteoclastogenesis and is dependent on osteoclast activity. Br J Haematol. 2002;116(2):278–90.
183. Croucher PI, Shipman CM, Lippitt J, et al. Osteoprotegerin inhibits the development of osteolytic bone disease in multiple myeloma. Blood. 2001;98(13):3534–40.
184. Vanderkerken K, De Leenheer E, Shipman C, et al. Recombinant osteoprotegerin decreases tumor burden and increases survival in a murine model of multiple myeloma. Cancer Res. 2003;63(2):287–9.

185. Kostenuik P, Nguyen H, McCabe J, et al. Denosumab, a fully human monoclonal antibody to RANKL, inhibits bone resorption and increases bone density in knock-in mice that express chimeric (murine/human) RANKL. J Bone Miner Res. 2009;24(2):182–95.

186. Body JJ, Facon T, Coleman RE, et al. A study of the biological receptor activator of nuclear factor-kappaB ligand inhibitor, denosumab, in patients with multiple myeloma or bone metastases from breast cancer. Clin Cancer Res. 2006;12(4):1221–8.

187. Yonemori K, Fujiwara Y, Minami H, et al. Phase 1 trial of denosumab safety, pharmacokinetics, and pharmacodynamics in Japanese women with breast cancer-related bone metastases. Cancer Sci. 2008;99(6):1237–42.

188. Vij R, Horvath N, Spencer A, Kitagawa K, et al. An open-label, Phase 2 trial of denosumab in the treatment of relapsed (R) or plateau-phase (PP) multiple myeloma (MM). Presented in the 49th ASH Annual Meeting and Exposition; 2007 Dec 8–11, Atlanta, GA.

189. Fizazi K, Lipton A, Mariette X, et al. Randomized phase II trial of denosumab in patients with bone metastases from prostate cancer, breast cancer, or other neoplasms after intravenous bisphosphonates. J Clin Oncol. 2009;27(10):1564–71.

190. Lipton A, Fizazi K, Stopeck AT, et al. Superiority of denosumab to zoledronic acid for prevention of skeletal-related events: a combined analysis of 3 pivotal, randomised, phase 3 trials. Eur J Cancer. 2012;48(16):3082–92.

191. Raje N, et al. Evaluating results from the multiple myeloma patient subset treated with denosumab or zoledronic acid in a randomized phase 3 trial. Blood Cancer J. 2016;6:e378.

192. Chantry AD, Heath D, Mulivor AW, et al. Inhibiting activin-A signaling stimulates bone formation and prevents cancer-induced bone destruction in vivo. J Bone Miner Res. 2010;25(12):2633–46.

193. Ruckle J, Jacobs M, Kramer W, et al. Single-dose, randomized, double-blind, placebo-controlled study of ACE-011 (ActRIIA-IgG1) in postmenopausal women. J Bone Miner Res. 2009;24(4):744–52.

194. Scullen T, Santo L, Vallet S, et al. Lenalidomide in combination with an activin A-neutralizing antibody: preclinical rationale for a novel anti-myeloma strategy. Leukemia. 2013;27(8):1715–21.

195. Oranger A, Carbone C, Izzo M, et al. Cellular mechanisms of multiple myeloma bone disease. Clin Dev Immunol. 2013;2013:289458.

196. Cao H, Zhu K, Qiu L, et al. Critical role of AKT protein in myeloma-induced osteoclast formation and osteolysis. J Biol Chem. 2013;288(42):30399–410.

197. Breitkreutz I, Raab MS, Vallet S, et al. Targeting MEK1/2 blocks osteoclast differentiation, function and cytokine secretion in multiple myeloma. Br J Haematol. 2007;139(1):55–63.

198. Tai YT, Landesman Y, Acharya C, et al. CRM1 inhibition induces tumor cell cytotoxicity and impairs osteoclastogenesis in multiple myeloma: molecular mechanisms and therapeutic implications. Leukemia. 2013;28(1):155–65.

199. Cafforio P, Savonarola A, Stucci S, et al. PTHrP produced by myeloma plasma cells regulates their survival and pro-osteoclast activity for bone disease progression. J Bone Miner Res. 2013;29(1):55–66.

200. Moreaux J, Hose D, Kassambara A, et al. Osteoclast-gene expression profiling reveals osteoclast-derived CCR2 chemokines promoting myeloma cell migration. Blood. 2011;117(4):1280–90.

201. Choi SJ, Oba Y, Gazitt Y, et al. Antisense inhibition of macrophage inflammatory protein 1-alpha blocks bone destruction in a model of myeloma bone disease. J Clin Invest. 2001;108(12):1833–41.

202. Roussou M, Tasidou A, Dimopoulos MA, et al. Increased expression of macrophage inflammatory protein-1alpha on trephine biopsies correlates with extensive bone disease, increased angiogenesis and advanced stage in newly diagnosed patients with multiple myeloma. Leukemia. 2009;23(11):2177–81.

203. Vallet S, Raje N, Ishitsuka K, et al. MLN3897, a novel CCR1 inhibitor, impairs osteoclastogenesis and inhibits the interaction of multiple myeloma cells and osteoclasts. Blood. 2007;110(10):3744–52.

204. Terpos E, Christoulas D, Papatheodorou A, et al. Dickkopf-1 is elevated in newly-diagnosed, symptomatic patients and in relapsed patients with multiple myeloma; correlations with

advanced disease features: a single-center experience in 284 patients. Presented in the 15th Congress of the European Hematology Association; 2010 June 10–13, Barcelona, Spain.

205. Steinman RM, Bonifaz L, Fujii S, et al. The innate functions of dendritic cells in peripheral lymphoid tissues. Adv Exp Med Biol. 2005;560:83–97.

206. Moester MJ, Papapoulos SE, CW L"w, et al. Sclerostin: current knowledge and future perspectives. Calcif Tissue Int. 2010;87(2):99–107.

207. Polyzos SA, Anastasilakis AD, Bratengeier C, et al. Serum sclerostin levels positively correlate with lumbar spinal bone mineral density in postmenopausal women—the six-month effect of risedronate and teriparatide. Osteoporos Int. 2012;23(3):1171–6.

208. Voskaridou E, Christoulas D, Plata E, et al. High circulating sclerostin is present in patients with thalassemia-associated osteoporosis and correlates with bone mineral density. Horm Metab Res. 2012;44(12):909–13.

209. Lewiecki EM. Sclerostin: a novel target for intervention in the treatment of osteoporosis. Discov Med. 2011;12(65):263–73.

210. von Metzler I, Krebbel H, Hecht M, et al. Bortezomib inhibits human osteoclastogenesis. Leukemia. 2007;21(9):2025–34.

211. Boissy P, Andersen TL, Lund T, et al. Pulse treatment with the proteasome inhibitor bortezomib inhibits osteoclast resorptive activity in clinically relevant conditions. Leuk Res. 2008;32(11):1661–8.

212. Terpos E, Heath DJ, Rahemtulla A, et al. Bortezomib reduces serum dickkopf-1 and receptor activator of nuclear factor-kappaB ligand concentrations and normalises indices of bone remodelling in patients with relapsed multiple myeloma. Br J Haematol. 2006;135(5):688–92.

213. Giuliani N, Morandi F, Tagliaferri S, et al. The proteasome inhibitor bortezomib affects osteoblast differentiation in vitro and in vivo in multiple myeloma patients. Blood. 2007;110(1):334–8.

214. Zangari M, Esseltine D, Lee CK, et al. Response to bortezomib is associated to osteoblastic activation in patients with multiple myeloma. Br J Haematol. 2005;131(1):71–3.

215. Heider U, Kaiser M, Muller C, et al. Bortezomib increases osteoblast activity in myeloma patients irrespective of response to treatment. Eur J Haematol. 2006;77(3):233–8.

216. Zangari M, Aujay M, Zhan F, et al. Alkaline phosphatase variation during carfilzomib treatment is associated with best response in multiple myeloma patients. Eur J Haematol. 2011;86(6):484–7.

217. Terpos E, Christoulas D, Kokkoris P, et al. Increased bone mineral density in a subset of patients with relapsed multiple myeloma who received the combination of bortezomib, dexamethasone and zoledronic acid. Ann Oncol. 2010;21(7):1561–2.

218. Terpos E, Kastritis E, Roussou M, et al. The combination of bortezomib, melphalan, dexamethasone and intermittent thalidomide is an effective regimen for relapsed/refractory myeloma and is associated with improvement of abnormal bone metabolism and angiogenesis. Leukemia. 2008;22(12):2247–56.

219. Terpos E, Christoulas D, Kastritis E, et al. VTD consolidation, without bisphosphonates, reduces bone resorption and is associated with a very low incidence of skeletal-related events in myeloma patients post-ASCT. Leukemia. 2013;28(4):928–34.

220. Delforge M, Terpos E, Richardson PG, et al. Fewer bone disease events, improvement in bone remodeling, and evidence of bone healing with Bortezomib plus melphalan-prednisone vs. melphalan-prednisone in the phase III VISTA trial in multiple myeloma. Eur J Haematol. 2011;86:372–84.

221. Terpos E, Mihou D, Szydlo R, et al. The combination of intermediate doses of thalidomide with dexamethasone is an effective treatment for patients with refractory/relapsed multiple myeloma and normalizes abnormal bone remodeling, through the reduction of sRANKL/osteoprotegerin ratio. Leukemia. 2005;19(11):1969–76.

222. Breitkreutz I, Raab MS, Vallet S, et al. Lenalidomide inhibits osteoclastogenesis, survival factors and bone-remodeling markers in multiple myeloma. Leukemia. 2008;22(10):1925–32.

223. Anderson G, Gries M, Kurihara N, et al. Thalidomide derivative CC-4047 inhibits osteoclast formation by down-regulation of PU.1. Blood. 2006;107(8):3098–105.

224. Bruzzese F, Pucci B, Milone MR, et al. Panobinostat synergizes with zoledronic acid in prostate cancer and multiple myeloma models by increasing ROS and modulating mevalonate and p38-MAPK pathways. Cell Death Dis. 2013;4:e878.
225. Bam R, Ling W, Khan S, et al. Role of Bruton's tyrosine kinase in myeloma cell migration and induction of bone disease. Am J Hematol. 2013;88(6):463–71.
226. Neri P, Kumar S, Fulciniti MT, et al. Neutralizing B-cell activating factor antibody improves survival and inhibits osteoclastogenesis in a severe combined immunodeficient human multiple myeloma model. Clin Cancer Res. 2007;13(19):5903–9.
227. Vanderkerken K, Medicherla S, Coulton L, et al. Inhibition of p38alpha mitogen-activated protein kinase prevents the development of osteolytic bone disease, reduces tumor burden, and increases survival in murine models of multiple myeloma. Cancer Res. 2007;67(10):4572–7.
228. Berenson J, Pflugmacher R, Jarzem P, et al. Balloon kyphoplasty versus non-surgical fracture management for treatment of painful vertebral body compression fractures in patients with cancer: a multicentre, randomised controlled trial. Lancet Oncol. 2011;12:225–3596.
229. Bouza C, Lopez-Cuadrado T, Cediel P, et al. Balloon kyphoplasty in malignant spinal fractures: a systematic review and meta-analysis. BMC Palliat Care. 2009;8:12.
230. McDonald RJ, Trout AT, Gray LA, et al. Vertebroplasty in multiple myeloma: outcomes in a large patient series. AJNR Am J Neuroradiol. 2008;29:642–8.
231. Huber F, McArthur N, Tanner M, et al. Kyphoplasty for patients with multiple myeloma is a safe surgical procedure: results from a large patient cohort. Clin Lymphoma Myeloma. 2009;9:375–80.
232. Zou J, Mei X, Gan M, et al. Kyphoplasty for spinal fractures from multiple myeloma. J Surg Oncol. 2010;102:43–7.
233. Dalbayrak S, Onen M, Yilmaz M, et al. Clinical and radiographic results of balloon kyphoplasty for treatment of vertebral body metastases and multiple myelomas. J Clin Neurosci. 2010;17:219–24.
234. Chew C, Craig L, Edwards R, et al. Safety and efficacy of percutaneous vertebroplasty in malignancy: a systematic review. Clin Radiol. 2011;66:63–72.
235. Buchbinder R, Osborne RH, Ebeling PR, et al. A randomized trial of vertebroplasty for painful osteoporotic vertebral fractures. N Engl J Med. 2009;361:557–68.
236. Kallmes DF, Comstock BA, Heagerty PJ, et al. A randomized trial of vertebroplasty for osteoporotic spinal fractures. N Engl J Med. 2009;361:569–79.
237. Bhargava A, Trivedi D, Kalva L, et al. Management of cancer-related vertebral compression fracture: comparison of treatment options: a literature meta-analysis. J Clin Oncol (Meeting Abstracts). 2009;27:e20529.
238. Rades D, Hoskin PJ, Stalpers LJ, et al. Short-course radiotherapy is not optimal for spinal cord compression due to myeloma. Int J Radiat Oncol Biol Phys. 2006;64:1452–7.
239. Hirsch AE, Jha RM, Yoo AJ, et al. The use of vertebral augmentation and external beam radiation therapy in the multimodal management of malignant vertebral compression fractures. Pain Physician. 2011;14:447–58.
240. Balducci M, Chiesa S, Manfrida S, et al. Impact of radiotherapy on pain relief and recalcification in plasma cell neoplasms: long-term experience. Strahlenther Onkol. 2011;187:114–9.
241. Price P, Hoskin PJ, Easton D, et al. Prospective randomised trial of single and multifraction radiotherapy schedules in the treatment of painful bony metastases. Radiother Oncol. 1986;6:247–55.
242. Mak KS, Lee LK, Mak RH, et al. Incidence and treatment patterns in hospitalizations for malignant spinal cord compression in the United States, 1998-2006. Int J Radiat Oncol Biol Phys. 2011;80:824–31.
243. Rades D, Veninga T, Stalpers LJ, et al. Outcome after radiotherapy alone for metastatic spinal cord compression in patients with oligometastases. J Clin Oncol. 2007;25:50–6.
244. Wedin R. Surgical treatment for pathologic fracture. Acta Orthop Scand Suppl. 2001;72(2p):1–29.
245. Utzschneider S, Schmidt H, Weber P, et al. Surgical therapy of skeletal complications in multiple myeloma. Int Orthop. 2011;35:1209–13.

Shaji Kumar

9.1 Introduction

Personalizing the treatment for a patient, or adapting the treatment for the individual patient, is a concept that is as old as the discipline of medicine. It is no wonder that one often comes across the reference to the "art" of medicine. A better understanding of the human physiology as well as disease biology has allowed us to inject more of science into the art of medicine, where decisions can be based more objectively on the scientific facts. The two basic requirements for such a personalized approach to treatment are a good understanding of the factors underlying disease heterogeneity and a choice of different treatment options that work in different ways. Even though there is increasing interest in incorporation of personalized medicine in oncology, limitations exist [1]. In the context of multiple myeloma (MM), both these basic requirements are increasingly becoming a reality, even though considerable amount of work remains to be done.

9.2 Disease Heterogeneity

As with many diseases, there is a considerable heterogeneity in the clinical presentation, response to treatment, and survival outcomes in MM [2]. Even though MM is often considered as one disease, characterized by clonal proliferation of mature plasma cells, it is increasingly becoming clear that this represents a group of disorders with a common phenotype, at least when visualized morphologically. The heterogeneity is composed of several features which can be broadly grouped into those that are tumor related and host specific and those resulting from differences in interaction between the tumor and host (Fig. 9.1) [3]. These characteristics can influence

S. Kumar, M.D.
Mayo Clinic, Rochester, MN, USA
e-mail: Kumar.Shaji@mayo.edu

© Springer International Publishing AG 2018   169
S.Z. Usmani, A.K. Nooka (eds.), *Personalized Therapy for Multiple Myeloma*,
https://doi.org/10.1007/978-3-319-61872-2_9

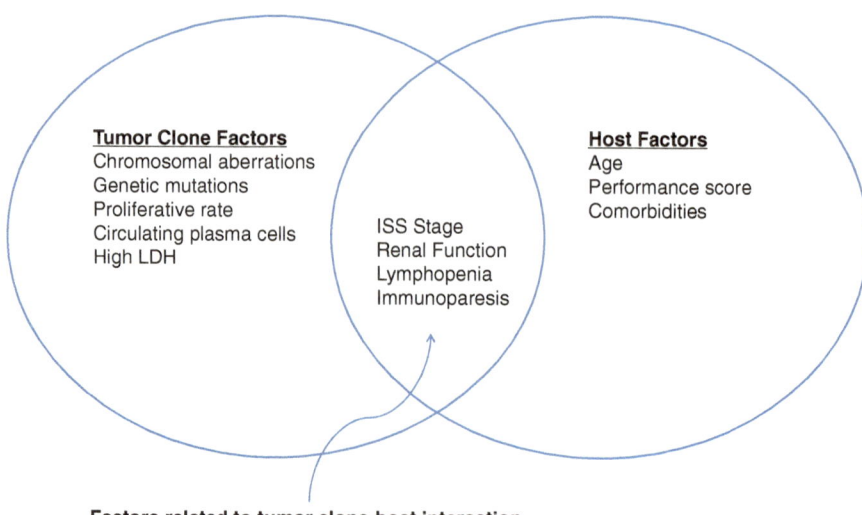

Tumor Clone Factors
Chromosomal aberrations
Genetic mutations
Proliferative rate
Circulating plasma cells
High LDH

ISS Stage
Renal Function
Lymphopenia
Immunoparesis

Host Factors
Age
Performance score
Comorbidities

Factors related to tumor clone-host interaction

Fig. 9.1 Complexity of risk stratification

the disease presentation in any given patient, may influence the treatment responses and toxicity to treatment, and the long-term outcomes including overall and disease-specific survival.

Tumor Characteristics

1. *Chromosomal abnormalities:* Much has been learned during the past decade regarding the spectrum of chromosomal abnormalities in myeloma, one of the most recognized and studied factors with respect to prognostic factors in MM [3–7]. Broadly, the abnormalities can be grouped into translocations involving the immunoglobulin heavy chain locus on chromosome 14 and a set of common partner chromosomes (chromosomes 4, 6, 8, 11, 16, and 20) or trisomies of several odd-numbered chromosomes (typically, 5, 7, 9, 15) or deletions (chromosome 1p, 17p, and 13q) or monosomies [13, 17]. The clinical outcomes associated with the presence of these abnormalities have been well studied, though the pathological mechanisms driven by these abnormalities are poorly understood. These chromosomal abnormalities can be observed across the entire spectrum of monoclonal gammopathies from MGUS to active myeloma, suggesting that the translocations and trisomies are early events in clonal evolution of the plasma cell [8, 9]. However, it remains unclear how it contributes to the disease progression across the spectrum. In addition to the differences in clinical outcomes, some phenotypic differences have been described and suggest that these abnormalities may allow us to further classify MM into related groups of diseases. Such a classification can be of clinical value if it predicts outcome but can be particularly relevant if it would allow us to select therapy. We are starting to see some early evidence regarding the utility of these markers in directing therapy. The first set of evidence came from early studies of the proteasome inhibitor

bortezomib, where it was clearly shown that the outcome of patients with deletion 13q could be improved by using bortezomib [10, 11]. Following this, several trials demonstrated a distinct benefit from using bortezomib in patients with t(4;14), another marker of poor outcome [11]. In particular, the early and continued use of bortezomib clearly improved the outcome of these patients compared with other treatment approaches. Patients with del17p, associated with loss of p53 gene, have one of the poorest outcomes among patients with MM. In this group of patients, the use of tandem autologous stem cell transplant followed by bortezomib maintenance, as well as the prolonged use of a PI/IMiD combination, appears to offer survival improvement [12]. More recently, ixazomib, an oral proteasome inhibitor, was shown to significantly negate the poor prognostic effect of del17p in a phase 3 trial in relapsed patients [13]. While it is not clear why specific treatment approaches may impact the outcome of these high-risk markers, recently described efficacy of targeted agents such as the bcl2 inhibitor venetoclax in t(11;14) MM has clear biological basis [14]. It appears that in MM with t(11;14), the plasma cells have a high ratio of bcl2 to mcl1, which increases the sensitivity of the MM cell to venetoclax. Another approach that takes into account the biology of the disease is ongoing trials with mdm2 inhibitors in combination with other myeloma agents, in patients with del17p, utilizing the mdm2 inhibition to increase the activity of the remaining p53 locus. These exciting findings, while still relatively preliminary, offer an avenue of clinical investigation for the development of therapies specifically targeted to the underlying biology of each chromosomal abnormality.

2. *Mutations*: Recent large-scale genomic evaluation of myeloma cells has shed light on the genetic complexity that underlies the entire spectrum of monoclonal gammopathies, with increasing heterogeneity accompanying disease progression [15–17]. While a large number of mutations have been described, including those that have been successfully targeted in other cancers, the most common mutations are still present in less than 5% pf patients. Two additional factors complicate the potential utility of these findings, the presence of multiple subclones with different sets of mutations as well as the constant waxing and waning of the different clones under pressure of specific therapeutic agents [18]. The prognostic value of these mutations still remains poorly understood, with some recent studies suggesting poor outcome associated with mutations involving p53 gene (often in conjunction with loss of one locus) and mutations involving the DNA repair genes [17]. The clinical relevance of these findings can be significant. The significant clonal evolution that is seen in the myeloma makes strong supporting argument for the use of drug combinations that can potentially lead to more comprehensive clonal eradication, though the direct data demonstrating this is lacking. The use of a PI/IMiD combination has been shown to be superior to IMiD alone in terms of overall survival, suggesting that the above assumption may be true [19]. Another implication of these finding is the potential to use targeted agents in myeloma, directed by identification of specific targetable mutations. Single patient reports have suggested that targeted agents such as the B-Raf inhibitor vemurafenib may have single agent activity in patients with

B-RafV600E mutation in their myeloma cells. However, these responses tend to be relatively short lasting given the clonal evolution and consequent escape. Clinical trials are being designed to examine the utility of such a mutation-driven treatment selection approach. Past experience suggests that this approach is more likely to be successful when the targeted agents are combined with other standard-of-care therapies, but this needs to be confirmed.

3. *Other tumor-related factors*: Several other tumor-related characteristics can be associated with poor outcome and can provide a window into the disease biology that can be targeted by specific approaches. High proliferative rate of plasma cells is often seen in conjunction with other poor prognostic factors and may warrant unique therapeutic approaches with specific classes of drugs [20–22]. Cell cycle-specific agents such as cdk inhibitors may have a unique role to play for these patients, especially in combination with other effective drugs, and need to be explored in clinical trials. While the presence of circulating plasma cells can be demonstrated during all disease stages, patients with myeloma with a significant number of circulating plasma cells, even when not fulfilling the definition of plasma cell leukemia, have inferior outcomes [23–25]. The underlying biology that permits these plasma cells to leave the conducive marrow microenvironment remains unclear, through a role for adhesion molecules have been proposed. These patients represent another group where specific treatment approaches need to be explored. While soft tissue plasmacytomas can present as isolated finding, when seen in conjunction with active myeloma it identifies patients with poor outcome. Systematic imaging with PET/CT at the time of diagnosis can detect plasmacytomas in less than 10% of patients; they are seen more often late in the disease course in the setting of relapsed and refractory disease [26]. Combination therapy, including those with conventional chemotherapy agents, is often employed to treat these late-stage patients with variable results. Elevated serum LDH is usually seen in conjunction with other markers of aggressive disease including high proliferative rates and extramedullary disease, and multidrug combinations such as VDT-PACE have often been used in these settings to gain disease control [6, 27]. The underlying biological drivers of these aggressive phenotypes remain poorly understood and should be the focus of systematic investigations if we are to succeed in improving disease outcomes.

Host Factors

1. *Age*: The median age at diagnosis of myeloma is 67–69 years in various series, and age continues to be a strong predictor of outcome despite the recent improvements in survival [28]. In fact, it has become clear that the older patient population may be deriving less benefit from the more recent improvements seen across myeloma [2]. Given no evidence to suggest that disease biology is significantly different in the older patient, the outcomes appear to be more related to the comorbidities and frailty that go with age and as described in more detail below. Age as a singular factor has been used for the longest time to make treatment decisions, and in fact many of the treatment algorithms often have this as the first

nodal point. The major reason for this approach has been the adoption of stem cell transplant in the initial management of myeloma. Many of the initial trials of stem cell transplant was limited to those below 65, though multiple non-randomized studies have shown that it is beneficial to the older patients as well. Adaptation of stem cell transplant to the older patients has involved either dose reduction of the conditioning chemotherapy or tandem transplant using half the dose of conditioning chemotherapy with each transplant. Instead of using chronological age as an absolute marker, it is more appropriate to consider this in the context of the frailty and other comorbidities as discussed below.

2. *Frailty*: Across all of cancers, there is increasing awareness of the relevance of patient frailty in determining the treatment strategy [29]. One of the best attempts at individualizing the treatment based on various measures of patient frailty has been put forth by the European investigators and has been widely adopted by the myeloma community. While complex measures of patient frailty such as the Charlson Comorbidity Index (CCI) allow better refinement of the patient status, simple assessments such as the Karnofsky Scale or the ECOG Performance Score can allow valuable stratification of patients that can be applied for treatment selection. The typical approach so far has been to modify the medication doses based on the measures of frailty, but there are two important question going forward: (1) can we develop multidrug combinations of newer agents which can be used safely with appropriate dose modifications, and (2) given the number of newer drugs and drug classes, are there specific drugs that have a favorable toxicity profile for the older patients? The former question is particularly relevant given the findings of better outcome with the combinations and the data regarding clonal evolution. In order to deliver multi-class drug combinations, we have to explore development of oral drugs and drug-dosing schedules that will minimize toxicity and reduce the care provider burden by reducing office visits while retaining the efficacy. Recent entrants to the drug armamentarium such as the monoclonal antibodies are well tolerated, and oral proteasome inhibitors will allow us to do exactly this.

3. *Comorbidities*: Given the older patient population, it is not surprising that a significant proportion of them will have serious comorbidities such as diabetes, hypertension, cardiac disease, as well as prior cancers among other illnesses. The impact of the myeloma medications on the control of these common disorders as well as drug interactions, given the polypharmacy involved, should be taken into consideration while making treatment decisions. Specific toxicities of commonly used drugs also should be taken into consideration while making treatment decisions. In particular, corticosteroids, a common ingredient of the current myeloma regimens, can have a deleterious impact on the diabetes control as well as hypertension, in addition to the usual side effects that can be magnified in the older patient. Acceleration of bone loss in the older patient with preexisting osteoporosis can significantly increase the risk of fractures. It is important to consider starting at lower doses in the older patients with careful monitoring and rapid dose reduction as required. Bortezomib can result in significant peripheral neuropathy and may worsen preexisting neuropathy related to diabetes.

Consideration should be given to the use of carfilzomib or ixazomib, both of which are associated with reduced risk of neuropathy. Cardiac toxicity can be seen with older drugs such as doxorubicin as well as newer drugs such as carfilzomib and can worsen preexisting cardiac failure, and careful evaluation prior to starting therapy and close monitoring during the treatment are very important. Adaptation of myeloma therapy to the elderly has been primarily empirical, and we certainly need well-controlled prospective trials to examine novel approaches for the older, frail patients.

Interaction of Host and Tumor

1. *ISS staging:* While both tumor-related characteristics as well as host characteristics are important factors in the disease management, the less predictable and less well-defined are the end results of the interaction between the host and the tumor that adds another dimension to the difficulty with individualizing treatments for myeloma. The commonly used International Staging System is a good example of the complex interaction between the tumor and host and is made up of two variables, namely, serum beta-2 microglobulin and serum albumin [30]. Serum B2M is an indirect measure of the tumor burden but can be affected by renal failure which can be the result of the paraprotein causing cast nephropathy or worsening preexisting nephropathy. Similarly, serum albumin can be lowered as a host reaction to the stress of a chronic illness such as myeloma through variety of mechanisms that have been identified. Patients with higher ISS stage have inferior outcome, but it is unclear how current therapies can be adapted to overcome the poor prognostic impact of this characteristic.

Implications of Response to Therapy

Characteristics of the disease at the time of presentation can provide guidance for selection of appropriate therapy, but the impact of the therapy employed can also be of great value in predicting subsequent disease course.

1. *Primary refractory disease*: Lack of response to initial therapy has become an uncommon phenomenon in myeloma with the introduction of the newer therapies, with less than 10% of patients failing to achieve at least a partial response to initial treatments, especially when drug combinations are used [31, 32]. Recent studies as well as studies prior to the introduction of the newer drugs had demonstrated a poor outcome for patients who fail the initial regimen employed. Newer drug combinations clearly reduce the proportion of these patients but, when observed, still predicts for very poor outcomes. Understanding the mechanism of primary refractoriness is critical to make gains in these patients. Prospective trials of primary refractory patients, especially those incorporating immune approaches, are clearly needed and will lead to improved outcomes.

2. *Early relapse*: Unlike the reduced incidence observed with primary refractory disease, over 20% of patients undergoing modern therapies relapse early, sometimes within a year, and the outcomes of these patients are very poor with overall survival of less than 2 years from the time of relapse [33–35]. These patients undergo multiple regimens with rapid development of resistance to all the current drugs, eventually succumbing to the disease. This group of patients along with those with primary refractory disease should be the focus of prospective clinical trials of novel regimens incorporating drugs with new mechanisms of action. These studies should be coupled with carefully designed correlative studies aimed at understanding the biological underpinnings of this clinical behavior. This remains a big gap in our current understanding, and progress in this area is vital to maintain the continued improvement of myeloma survival.

3. *Depth of response and MRD status*: Adapting treatment based on the observed response has not been a major focus a decade ago where a limited armamentarium of drugs and most treatment approaches prescribed a limited duration of therapy followed by observation. Recent improvements in measurement of the depth of response (aka residual tumor burden), deeper responses with the newer regimens, increasing adoption of the concept of continued response, increasing drug options, and the rising cost of the new drugs all have brought the concept of response-adapted therapy into the limelight. Recent efforts at developing consensus criteria for defining MRD status in MM have also propelled this area to the forefront of current investigations [36]. Studies, so far, including meta-analysis of prospective trials, clearly show improved overall survival among patients achieving an MRD negative status with various therapies, clearly demonstrating its role as a surrogate endpoint for assessment of therapeutic efficacy [37, 38]. However, the clinical utility of this marker remains to be validated in prospective clinical trials. The opportunities for potential clinical applications are many. The most important areas for MRD application include decisions on changing therapy for lack of MRD negativity and limiting duration of therapy based on MRD status. The former is particularly relevant in the context of high-risk MM, where failure to achieve MRD negativity appears to be a harbinger of early relapse. The ability to stop therapy based on MRD assessment also has implications on the overall cost of myeloma therapy as well as the potential long-term toxicity of the currently used drugs. Another important aspect of future investigation will be the development of less invasive and more sensitive techniques of residual disease assessment such as those based on circulating cell-free DNA and or circulating cells.

9.2.1   Challenges to Individualizing Therapy in MM

Individualized or personalized medicine is clearly the buzz word for the twenty-first century, and may mean different things to different people. The ability to customize therapy to provide the maximum duration of disease control with the least toxicity, based on factors that drive disease heterogeneity, remains the bedrock of this

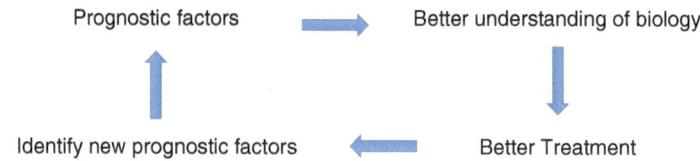

Fig. 9.2 Improving prognostication in MM

concept. By definition it is dynamic, as customization to successfully account for certain disease characteristics will make those features less relevant and will lead to identification of other disease characteristics which then will account for disease heterogeneity (Fig. 9.2). This in turn will require further customization based on studies into disease biology and prospective treatment trials. Rather than considering this negatively, it should be the incentive for continued work aimed at improving the disease outcomes, which at some point will translate to a cure for this disease.

References

1. Tannock IF, Hickman JA. Limits to personalized cancer medicine. N Engl J Med. 2016;375:1289–94.
2. Kumar SK, Dispenzieri A, Lacy MQ, et al. Continued improvement in survival in multiple myeloma: changes in early mortality and outcomes in older patients. Leukemia. 2014;28:1122–8.
3. Chng WJ, Dispenzieri A, Chim CS, et al. IMWG consensus on risk stratification in multiple myeloma. Leukemia. 2014;28:269–77.
4. Boyd KD, Ross FM, Chiecchio L, et al. A novel prognostic model in myeloma based on co-segregating adverse FISH lesions and the ISS: analysis of patients treated in the MRC myeloma IX trial. Leukemia. 2012;26:349–55.
5. Jacobus SJ, Kumar S, Uno H, et al. Impact of high-risk classification by FISH: an Eastern Cooperative Oncology Group (ECOG) study E4A03. Br J Haematol. 2011;155(3):340–8.
6. Palumbo A, Avet-Loiseau H, Oliva S, et al. Revised international staging system for multiple myeloma: a report from International Myeloma Working Group. J Clin Oncol. 2015;33(26):2863–9.
7. Kumar S, Fonseca R, Ketterling RP, et al. Trisomies in multiple myeloma: impact on survival in patients with high-risk cytogenetics. Blood. 2012;119:2100–5.
8. Rajkumar SV, Gupta V, Fonseca R, et al. Impact of primary molecular cytogenetic abnormalities and risk of progression in smoldering multiple myeloma. Leukemia. 2013;27:1738–44.
9. Chng WJ, Van Wier SA, Ahmann GJ, et al. A validated FISH trisomy index demonstrates the hyperdiploid and nonhyperdiploid dichotomy in MGUS. Blood. 2005;106:2156–61. doi:10.1182/blood-2005-02-0761.
10. Jagannath S, Richardson PG, Sonneveld P, et al. Bortezomib appears to overcome the poor prognosis conferred by chromosome 13 deletion in phase 2 and 3 trials. Leukemia. 2007;21:151–7.
11. Avet-Loiseau H, Leleu X, Roussel M, et al. Bortezomib plus dexamethasone induction improves outcome of patients with t(4;14) myeloma but not outcome of patients with del(17p). J Clin Oncol. 2010;28:4630–4.
12. Neben K, Lokhorst HM, Jauch A, et al. Administration of bortezomib before and after autologous stem cell transplantation improves outcome in multiple myeloma patients with deletion 17p. Blood. 2012;119:940–8.

13. Moreau P, Masszi T, Grzasko N, et al. Oral ixazomib, lenalidomide, and dexamethasone for multiple myeloma. N Engl J Med. 2016;374:1621–34.
14. Touzeau C, Le Gouill S, Mahe B, et al. Deep and sustained response after venetoclax therapy in a patient with very advanced refractory myeloma with translocation t(11;14). Haematologica. 2017;102(3):e112–4.
15. Chapman MA, Lawrence MS, Keats JJ, et al. Initial genome sequencing and analysis of multiple myeloma. Nature. 2011;471:467–72.
16. Egan JB, Shi CX, Tembe W, et al. Whole-genome sequencing of multiple myeloma from diagnosis to plasma cell leukemia reveals genomic initiating events, evolution, and clonal tides. Blood. 2012;120:1060–6.
17. Walker BA, Boyle EM, Wardell CP, et al. Mutational spectrum, copy number changes, and outcome: results of a sequencing study of patients with newly diagnosed myeloma. J Clin Oncol. 2015;33(33):3911–20.
18. Keats JJ, Chesi M, Egan JB, et al. Clonal competition with alternating dominance in multiple myeloma. Blood. 2012;120(5):1067–76.
19. Andrulis M, Lehners N, Capper D, et al. Targeting the BRAF V600E mutation in multiple myeloma. Cancer Discov. 2013;3:862–9.
20. Morice WG II, Timm MM, Jevremovic D, Ketterling RP, Kumar S, Reichard KK. Plasma cell phenotyping and DNA content analysis by 8-color flow cytometry: a highly sensitive assay that simultaneously measures clonality, ploidy, and proliferation. Mod Pathol. 2013;26:349A–50A.
21. Hose D, Reme T, Hielscher T, et al. Proliferation is a central independent prognostic factor and target for personalized and risk-adapted treatment in multiple myeloma. Haematologica. 2011;96:87–95.
22. Kumar S, Timm M, Lacy M, et al. Combining measurements of plasma cell apoptosis and proliferation in multiple myeloma identifies patients with poor survival. Blood. 2005;106:952A.
23. Gonsalves WI, Rajkumar SV, Gupta V, et al. Quantification of clonal circulating plasma cells in newly diagnosed multiple myeloma: implications for redefining high-risk myeloma. Leukemia. 2014;28:2060–5.
24. Gonsalves WI, Morice WG, Rajkumar V, et al. Quantification of clonal circulating plasma cells in relapsed multiple myeloma. Br J Haematol. 2014;167:500–5.
25. Kumar S, Rajkumar SV, Kyle RA, et al. Prognostic value of circulating plasma cells in monoclonal gammopathy of undetermined significance. J Clin Oncol. 2005;23:5668–74.
26. Usmani SZ, Heuck C, Mitchell A, et al. Extramedullary disease portends poor prognosis in multiple myeloma and is over-represented in high-risk disease even in the era of novel agents. Haematologica. 2012;97:1761–7.
27. Barlogie B, Smallwood L, Smith T, Alexanian R. High serum levels of lactic dehydrogenase identify a high-grade lymphoma-like myeloma. Ann-Intern-Med. 1989;110:521–5.
28. Ludwig H, Bolejack V, Crowley J, et al. Survival and years of life lost in different age cohorts of patients with multiple myeloma. J Clin Oncol. 2010;28:1599–605.
29. Palumbo A, Bringhen S, Ludwig H, et al. Personalized therapy in multiple myeloma according to patient age and vulnerability: a report of the European Myeloma Network (EMN). Blood. 2011;118:4519–29.
30. Greipp PR, San Miguel J, Durie BG, et al. International staging system for multiple myeloma. J Clin Oncol. 2005;23:3412–20.
31. Majithia N, Vincent Rajkumar S, Lacy MQ, et al. Outcomes of primary refractory multiple myeloma and the impact of novel therapies. Am J Hematol. 2015;90:981–5.
32. Parrish C, Rahemtulla A, Cavet J, et al. Autologous stem cell transplantation is an effective salvage therapy for primary refractory multiple myeloma. Biol Blood Marrow Transplant. 2015;21:1330–4.
33. Jimenez-Zepeda VH, Reece DE, Trudel S, Chen C, Tiedemann R, Kukreti V. Early relapse after single auto-SCT for multiple myeloma is a major predictor of survival in the era of novel agents. Bone Marrow Transplant. 2015;50:204–8.

34. Majithia N, Rajkumar SV, Lacy MQ, et al. Early relapse following initial therapy for multiple myeloma predicts poor outcomes in the era of novel agents. Leukemia. 2016;30:2208–13.
35. Venner CP, Connors JM, Sutherland HJ, et al. Novel agents improve survival of transplant patients with multiple myeloma including those with high-risk disease defined by early relapse (<12 months). Leuk Lymphoma. 2011;52:34–41.
36. Kumar S, Paiva B, Anderson KC, et al. International Myeloma Working Group consensus criteria for response and minimal residual disease assessment in multiple myeloma. Lancet Oncol. 2016;17:e328–46.
37. Munshi NC, Avet-Loiseau H, Rawstron AC, et al. Association of minimal residual disease with superior survival outcomes in patients with multiple myeloma: a meta-analysis. JAMA Oncol. 2017;3:28–35.
38. Paiva B, Garcia-Sanz R, San Miguel JF. Multiple myeloma minimal residual disease. Cancer Treat Res. 2016;169:103–22.